Back Pain

A Practical Guide to Coping

Linda and David Tagg

The Crowood Press

First published in 1989 by
The Crowood Press
Ramsbury, Marlborough
Wiltshire SN8 2HE

© Linda and David Tagg 1989

All rights reserved. No part of this publication may be
reproduced or transmitted in any form or by any means,
electronic or mechanical, including photocopy, recording, or
any information storage and retrieval system without
permission in writing from the publishers.

British Library Cataloguing in Publication Data

Tagg, David
Back pain: a practical guide to coping
1. Man. Back. Backache. Therapy
I. Title II. Tagg, Linda
616.7'3068

ISBN 1 85223 161 0

Dedication

To Audrey, Maurice and Dorothy, our parents, and Carol

Picture Credits

Line illustrations by Claire Upsdale-Jones

Typeset by Inforum Typesetting, Portsmouth
Printed in Great Britain by MacLehose & Partners Ltd, Portsmouth

Contents

Introduction 5
1 The Causes of Back Pain 7
2 Your Back – the Basic Structure 8
3 What Can Go Wrong 18
4 Reducing the Stress 25
5 Coping with Back Pain 58
6 Treatments Available 70
Appendix – Useful Addresses 96

Acknowledgements

A publication of this kind would not be possible without the knowledge we have gained from various persons and publications, either knowingly or unknowingly; to any whose name we have inadvertently omitted, our sincere apologies.

For reading parts of the manuscript our thanks go to Dr T P Nash, Consultant Anaesthetist and Director of Pain Relief Services, and Mr R S Browne, Consultant Orthopaedic Surgeon.

For information on back care in motherhood, Mrs Jayne Potter, Chartered Physiotherapist.

For valuable help in typing the manuscript, Mrs Audrey Norford.

For research material, A Nachemson, C R Hayne, D A Stubbs, J D G Troup, J J Keegan, P H Newman, The Back Pain Association, and The Robens Institute, University of Surrey.

To our patients, our thanks for encouraging us to continue our fight against back pain.

Introduction

THE PRESENT BACK PAIN PROBLEM

The back pain problem in Great Britain is a big one, and figures show that it is getting worse rather than better. The latest statistics available, based on figures from 1982, show that the number of working days lost due to back pain actually exceeds those lost due to action taken in industrial disputes. Lost production due to sickness through back pain has been calculated to exceed £1,018 million each year. Payments that are now being made annually by the DHSS to sufferers of back pain are said to be in excess of £193 million.

More importantly, and coming a lot closer to home, the quality of your personal life will be greatly affected if you become a sufferer, as those of you who do suffer with back pain will already know.

Perhaps the most frightening statistic of all is that four out of every five people in Great Britain will suffer from back pain to some extent, at some time during their life.

The purpose of this book is to help you to reduce the risk of injuring your back, if you do not yet have a back pain problem. If unfortunately you do suffer, the book will help you to reduce the risk of aggravating or creating a reoccurrence of your condition, and will give you an insight into some of the ways in which back pain can now be managed. In this way we hope that the amount of pain or discomfort that you have been experiencing can, perhaps, be reduced.

Whether you suffer from back pain, or are trying to avoid developing a serious back problem, the amount that you gain from this book is down to you. There is plenty of useful

Introduction

advice and information on what can go wrong and how the stress on your back can be reduced. There are tips on how to cope with an attack of back pain, however slight, but only you can put these into practice, and it will not be easy.

You will probably find that you have to change the habits of a lifetime, which you will not, of course, be able to achieve overnight. It will involve taking time and effort on your part to start thinking about your back and your body shape whenever you do anything, and whatever you do. But always remember that it is *your* back, and *you* are the one that is going to suffer the pain and discomfort if your back pain develops. With determination over the next few months, you can help to improve your quality of life and reduce the risk of creating further back problems.

THE INDIVIDUALITY OF BACK PAIN

It is often very difficult with back pain to make a precise diagnosis as to exactly which structure or structures within the back are causing the pain. Sometimes, having listened to a patient talking about their particular pain, and having examined them, it is possible to say, yes, you have damaged this disc or that ligament. However, on many occasions one cannot be at all certain what the precise cause of the pain being experienced is.

For this reason it is important to listen to your own back, and its feelings. Try out some of the suggestions in the following pages, and use the ones that suit you as an individual. You will soon know if you are attempting to do something that your back does not like, or is harmful to you, because your back will tell you; it will start to cause you pain.

1
The Causes of Back Pain

The Robens Institute at Surrey University, England has undertaken considerable research into the back pain problem. During their research, they have found that it is not primarily heavy lifting that causes back pain, as is widely believed, but more the poor postures that we are sometimes forced to take up regularly for prolonged periods of time.

As we have become more and more 'civilised', a wonderfully mechanised world has been built up to help us to carry out all sorts of tasks, at work, in the home, and also in our leisure pursuits. However, more and more people are now beginning to realise that much equipment has been designed primarily to do a job, with little thought as to how the user's body will fit it, or what shape the body will have to adopt in order to use it. So, we often take up poor postures in many activities during our daily lives. This poor posture will have a build-up effect over the months and years, slowly weakening the various structures of the spine, until one day, something 'goes' and your back pain problem has begun.

Ergonomics is a growing science. In this science pieces of equipment are not only designed to fulfil a function, but also so that they fit the human being that will be using them. Ergonomically-designed equipment and pieces of furniture are becoming more common, and more companies are now employing ergonomists to look at the designs in the workplace.

It will obviously be many years before all the equipment and furniture that is available to the majority of people is ergonomically designed, but there is usually something that you can alter now in order to achieve a safer and improved posture.

2
Your Back – The Basic Structure

In order to be able to understand our back: what can go wrong with it; what sort of things cause our various aches and pains; and what we can do to alleviate any problems we may experience; it is essential that we have some kind of knowledge of how the back is constructed and how it works.

The back, or spine, is made up of a column of individual, irregularly-shaped small bones called vertebrae. In between each of these vertebrae are found the discs (*see* Fig 1).

With all the vertebrae and discs in their correct position and shape, the spine is curved in an 'S' shape (*see* Fig 2).

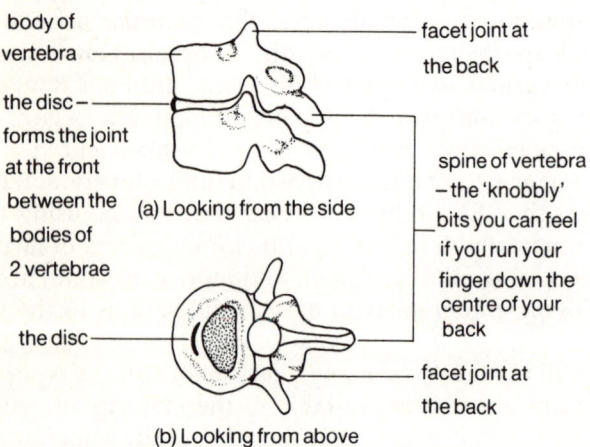

Fig 1   The spinal unit.

Your Back – The Basic Structure

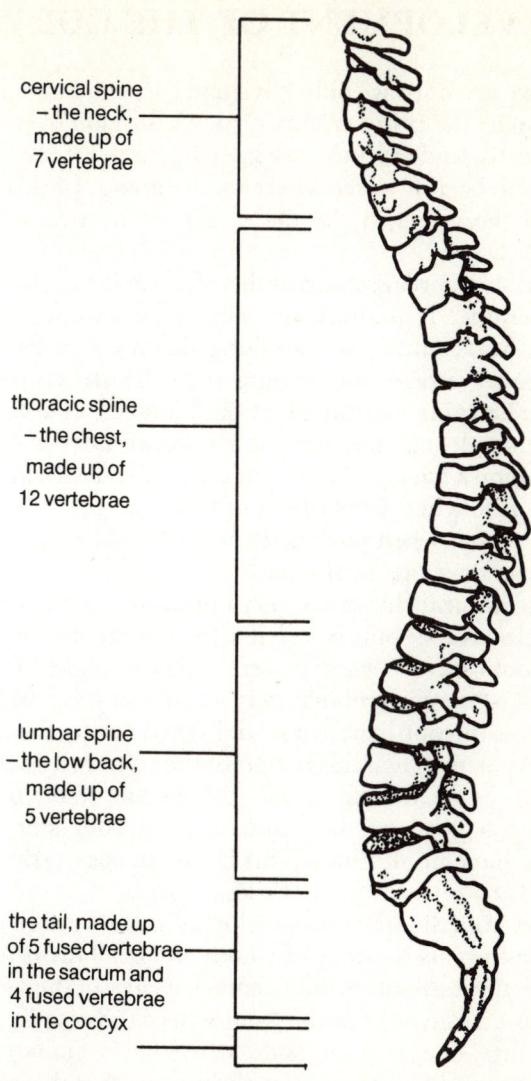

cervical spine – the neck, made up of 7 vertebrae

thoracic spine – the chest, made up of 12 vertebrae

lumbar spine – the low back, made up of 5 vertebrae

the tail, made up of 5 fused vertebrae in the sacrum and 4 fused vertebrae in the coccyx

Fig 2 The 'S' shaped spine.

Your Back – The Basic Structure

DEVELOPMENT OF THE CURVES

When we are born we only have one curve in our spine; this is known as the primary curve. As we develop over the first few months, and start to crawl, we begin to lift our head up in order to be able to see where we are going. In this way we develop the curve in the neck, one of the two secondary curves.

You may not realise that at this stage in life, a child's back is vulnerable. If parents are over-eager to encourage the child to walk and it keeps falling down on to its bottom, unnecessary stress can be put on to the structures of the spine. The spine can therefore be damaged at a very early age, although this may not show up until later in life when you develop a back problem. For some of you with back pain, this may be when your problem first started.

Eventually, when your body is ready for you to walk the last curve develops in the back.

These natural curves are very important to the strength of our backs, as the spine is ten times as strong, in comparison, as it would have been if it were poker-straight. You may, perhaps, sometimes notice that when you have back pain, the curves in your back are straightened out by the action of muscle spasm. When this happens, the spine loses some of its strength. It is, therefore, very important that you try to maintain a good posture, and to keep your spine in the correct shape at all times. This is not an easy task, but one that will be rewarding in the long run.

Apart from the spine supporting us in our upright posture, it also allows us to move our body about. This is achieved because there are three joints between each of the vertebrae. There is a large joint at the front where the disc is, and two little joints, one on either side at the back, known as facet joints. If we add all of these up this means that there are over seventy joints in the spine. That's a very large number of joints in your back which can be damaged in one way or another, just as easily as you can sprain an ankle. Now, the amount of movement possible between any two of the vertebrae is very small, but when you add up all the movement between all the vertebrae, and think of what some people can do with their spine, there's quite a large range of movement available.

THE DISC

The joint at the front is formed by the disc, sitting between two of the vertebrae. Basically, the disc's structure is made up of cartilage, which is the smooth, shiny white substance that you see on the end of a bone from a joint of meat. The cartilage forms a stringy ring on the outside of the disc with a squashy middle containing a watery substance. Each of these discs between the vertebrae of the spine acts as a shock absorber, to protect us. During our everyday activities, when we're walking around and running up and down stairs, there is a certain amount of jarring force that travels up from our feet through the bones of our bodies. Now, if this jarring force was allowed to travel right up to the top bone in the body, the skull, then the shaking of our brains would not do us a lot of good! So the discs in our spines are designed to absorb the shock wave as it travels upwards toward the head.

The lowest disc in the spine absorbs a certain amount of the shock wave, and spreads it out sideways. The rest travels up to the next disc where a bit more of the shock is absorbed and spread out, and so on right up to the top of the spine. So by the time it reaches the skull, the shock wave is very much reduced and is unlikely to do us any permanent harm.

However, this means that the lowest disc always takes the maximum shock wave which is one reason why the lower back tends to be one of the biggest problem areas of the spine. Having said this, it is important to look after the whole

Your Back – The Basic Structure

of your spine, and not to think about the back as being the lower back only. Always remember that your back goes right from your head at the top, down to your tail at the bottom, and it is essential that you look after all of it. If you do already have a problem at one end of your spine, then you are much more likely to develop a problem at the other end. Remember that the spine is made up of individual vertebrae, jointed together, and that if you move one end, you will have some effect at the other end.

During the day, as we are involved in the normal activities of sitting, standing and walking around, the watery substance in the squashy middle of the disc is gradually squeezed out because of the pressure that we are putting on the discs. This is absorbed into the bones above and below.

At night, when we lie down to sleep, the pressure is taken off the discs, the fluid is reabsorbed into it and it swells back to its normal thickness. If you measure yourself first thing in the morning when you get up, and then measure yourself last thing at night before you lie down, you will probably find that you are a bit shorter by the end of the day because the disc has lost some of its water content. For those of you who drive, you may well have noticed that when you get into your car in the morning, you have to adjust your driving mirrors, and when you get back in at the end of the day, you have to adjust them again. This is because the spine has 'shrunk' by about ¾ in (2cm), as the squashy middle has been pushed out during the day.

The importance of this is that when the fluid of the squashy middle has been squeezed out, the disc becomes more brittle, and is therefore more likely to become damaged or torn. So you are more likely to damage your discs at the end of the working day than at the start.

As we get older, the amount of water content in the disc becomes less and less. This is a natural part of the ageing process and happens to all of us, like grey hair and wrinkles, and can happen sooner in life with some people than it does with others. So, the older you get the less effective the discs become as shock absorbers, and the more likely you are to be at risk of damaging them.

Certain postures and shapes that we put our bodies into, exert more pressure on the discs than others. Looking at the three basic positions of sitting, standing and lying, it has been shown by research that sitting puts the most pressure on to the discs. This explains why it is that if someone is suffering from a disc problem, they often cannot sit down at all, because of the pain that it creates. On the other hand, lying flat puts the least amount of pressure on to the disc. So if you are caught lying down, you can always use the excuse that it's purely for medicinal purposes!

LIGAMENTS AND MUSCLES

Ligaments are essentially very tough pieces of gristle. They are tough, non-elastic pieces of tissue, designed to hold everything together and keep everything in place. There are many ligaments involved in the structure of the spine, at the front, at the back, down each side, and even through the hole in each vertebra.

The muscles around the spine have two main functions. First, they allow us the ability to move our spines around in the way we do. Secondly, they support our bodies in the upright posture, maintaining our naturally-developed 'S' shaped curve.

However, if we develop a bad or poor posture, then the muscles are continually having to work to try and keep us upright. When these muscles are working like this, then they are continually using up unnecessary energy, making you feel quite tired by the end of the day. Also, when a muscle works it shortens, which puts additional pressure on the discs. This will tend to increase the ageing process of the disc, and will also increase any pain being experienced.

Your Back – The Basic Structure

THE ABDOMINAL BALLOON

One of the body's built-in reflexes is the abdominal balloon. If we put any pressure on our spine, such as by lifting or pushing something, then the abdominal balloon comes into play automatically to protect us.

How does it work? Just imagine for a moment your abdominal cavity as a round balloon, with the muscles of your pelvis underneath it and your spinal column behind it. Above it is the large diaphragm muscle which separates your chest from your abdominal cavity. In front of it you have your abdominal or tummy muscles.

If we lean forward or begin to handle anything, the weight of our trunk will make us fall forward unless something happens to maintain us in an upright position. To prevent us from falling, the muscles at the bottom of the spine start working to keep us upright. Because they are attached to either end of the spine, they put pressure on the structures of the spine, as they shorten, creating stress. In response to this, the body automatically contracts the abdominal muscles which changes the balloon's shape. It then becomes sausage-shaped, pushing down against the pelvic floor, and up against the diaphragm. With this sausage-shaped balloon pushing in opposite directions at each end, the structures of the spine are pushed apart slightly, and the stress going through the spine can be reduced by up to twenty-five per cent.

So our balloon is a very useful gadget to have. But, like any balloon, it can burst, meaning that you're likely to suffer a hernia if you're male, or a prolapse if you're female. To reduce the risk of your abdominal balloon bursting, you should ensure that you do two things. First, make sure that your abdominal and pelvic floor muscles are nice and strong. Secondly, don't hold your breath when your balloon is working but breathe out like weight lifters do. Whether you are pushing, lifting or just exercising your abdominal muscles, make sure that you either breathe normally, or, if you find this difficult, as you do the exercise or take the strain, breathe out.

Something else that you will see weight lifters doing is wearing a belt whilst doing the lift. A belt, whether it be a surgical belt, corset, pantie girdle or just tight jeans, can enhance the effect of your balloon, making it work that much more effectively. But beware of wearing something like this on a regular basis, for long periods, as it allows your tummy muscles to 'go on holiday' as they have no work to do. As a result of this they will become very weak and when you take the belt off, your back will then have no support from the abdominal balloon. You end up with a worse problem than you started with. So a corset or a belt can be very useful for putting on for particular occasions when you are going to be stressing your spine, for example, when gardening. But be very wary of wearing one on a permanent basis. We have seen a number of patients over the years whose back pain has been due purely to weak tummy muscles. Strengthen these and the back pain has gone, without resorting to any other form of treatment.

It is worth noting that if you are reaching or lifting above shoulder level, your balloon cannot work. This is because, in this position, you put your tummy muscles on the stretch, and when stretched they can't work. Therefore, working in this posture you will have one hundred per cent of the stress going through your spine, while the little facet joints are being crunched together by you leaning backwards. So, do try to avoid lifting and reaching above shoulder level if at all possible. Find something suitable to stand on which allows you to adopt a better position.

LEVERAGE ON THE SPINE

The spine can be seen as very much like a crane jib when considering the forces of leverage. In the position shown in

Your Back – The Basic Structure

Fig 3, the load or weight is being handled a long way from the base. The forces of leverage make this a very unstable position, and it won't take much of an increase in weight before the whole thing topples over, or something is damaged. In Fig 4, the weight is being handled much closer to the base. This position is far more stable, and a greater load can be handled with less danger of damage occurring. Modern cranes have lights or buzzers to warn that they are being overloaded, to prevent the operator damaging an expensive piece of equipment. What warning sign do we humans have? That's right. Pain! But by then it's too late, the damage has been done and quite possibly, permanently. This is why it is so important to get into the habit of keeping your back in a good natural posture and to avoid stooping. This way you reduce to a minimum the risk of anything snapping.

Many people in the past have said to us, 'It's all very well, but I haven't the time to think of all this.' As we said right at

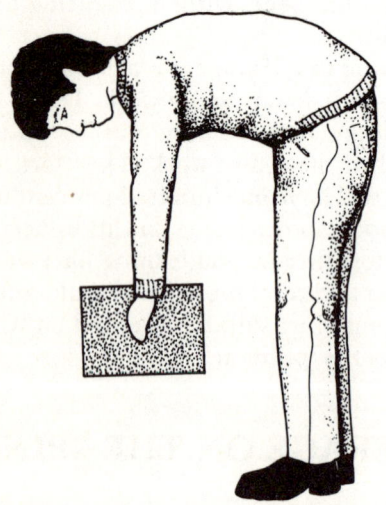

Fig 3 The unstable lifting position.

Your Back – The Basic Structure

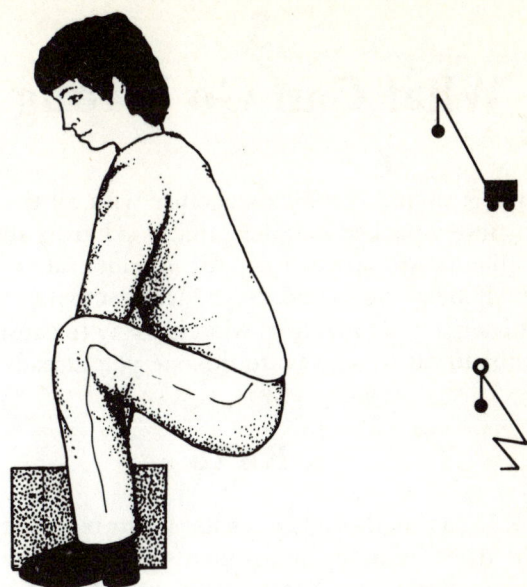

Fig 4   The stable lifting position.

the beginning, it will take time and effort on your part. But if you think about your back, and the shapes you adopt during certain activities, you will begin to change. Eventually you will find that you end up with a new set of habits, and no matter how busy you are, you will automatically adopt the best posture for the activity in which you are involved. By this time things will take no longer, but you'll be a lot safer.

3
What Can Go Wrong

The spine is such a complex structure with all the various parts so closely packed together, that it is hardly surprising that problems will arise if we do not look after it. This chapter will help you to understand what activities to avoid, and to become more aware of what is likely to cause a back pain problem, or to aggravate the one you already have.

X-RAYS

When an X-ray is taken, it only shows your bones. It doesn't show the discs, muscles or ligaments. Many patients with back pain will have an X-ray taken, and then be told that everything appears normal. This does not mean that the pain is an imaginary one, just that the pain is not originating from the bones in your back. This is the case with most people, so don't be surprised. It is not the bones producing the pain, but the soft tissues, such as the discs, muscles and ligaments, which don't show up on the X-ray.

Although you cannot see a disc on the X-ray, you can see the space that it occupies. If the discs are showing signs of ageing, they lose their water content, and consequently do not take up as much space. This will show up on the X-ray as a narrowing of the disc space. Anyone over the age of thirty is likely to show signs of the lowest disc wearing out. The reason for this is that the lowest disc takes the maximum jarring effect from everyday activities such as walking and running. The term used to describe this natural ageing of the discs is spondylosis and it comes to us all eventually. But having worn out discs does not necessarily mean that you

What Can Go Wrong

will suffer pain. There are many people walking about with what could be described as 'grotty' X-rays, showing a lot of aged discs, but they don't have any pain. It's what you do on top of this wearing out process that will give rise to pain, such as – doing a lot of stooping, twisting and jerky movements, or putting excessive vibrations through your spine.

THE EFFECT OF STOOPING

Stooping (*see* Fig 5) poses one of our biggest problems in life. Although you may feel no pain or discomfort whatever when you stoop forward, everything at the back of the spine is being stretched. All the muscles and ligaments running down the back of the spine may be stretched too much, and as a result they can tear. It is this tearing which will give rise to aches and pains.

The little facet joints at either side of the back of the spine are being stretched apart. By overstretching these joints you

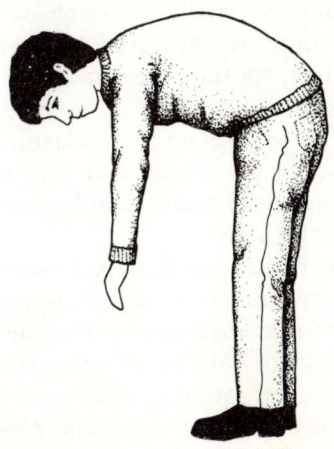

Fig 5   The stoop.

What Can Go Wrong

can sprain any one of them, in just the same way that you can sprain an ankle. Then you will feel pain.

When the disc is stretched at the back, part of the stringy ring may tear and move. When you are stooping forward, as well as stretching everything at the back, you are also exerting pressure on the front of the disc. This pressure can cause the squashy middle to be pushed out backwards. This is what we know as the 'slipped disc'. It is not the whole disc shunting out of place one way or the other, but when you have damaged the disc and a piece of the stringy ring tears and moves, the squashy middle is pushed out backwards, or you may get a combination of the two.

Many people do plenty of stooping and don't have any pain (giving rise to the 'It won't happen to me' syndrome), but just think back to exactly how your back problem first started. Most people say things like 'I wasn't lifting anything, I just bent forward to pick a cup off the table, and suddenly I had this awful pain in my back; I couldn't move'. Or: 'Well, it just slowly built up; gradually got worse; I can't think of any particular reason why'. Quite simply, the reason why is that everytime we stoop, although we feel no pain whatsoever at the time, we are gradually weakening the structures down. Then, one day, eventually something 'goes' and back pain begins.

Our ligaments can be likened to an elastic band in that they will take so much stretching, and then suddenly one goes 'ping'. It is when one or more of our ligaments 'pings' or tears that we get sudden pain.

A disc can be likened to a grape, in that you can squeeze a grape at one end a few times and nothing appears to happen; squeeze it again, and the skin at the back suddenly tears and out comes the pulp. With our disc, it is the stringy ring that tears, and out comes the squashy middle.

This is why it is *so* important to get into good habits and try to avoid stooping. Stooping feels fine until you get pain, but by then it is too late – the damage is done.

TWISTING

If you keep your feet and legs still when you are standing or sitting, and twist your body around to look at something behind you, you will be putting a nasty shearing strain on to the structures of the spine. In comparison, it's a bit like getting hold of a carrot at both ends and twisting it to break it in half. There will be a certain amount of twist movement but eventually something has to give, and damage occurs.

A particularly nasty position to get your body into is to stoop over, and then twist to the side and pick something up. This 'body shape' puts a very heavy strain on a weak part of the disc. Many people who have very nasty back problems are those who have stooped over, twisted to one side and then tried to lift something. But this is quite a common thing for people to do during the day. We go to open a cupboard or refrigerator door, and rather than walk round to the front, we open the door so that it is in front of our legs and we then stoop over and twist to reach in and get something out. One day it could be the cause of very severe pain.

VIBRATION

Most people have heard of the ability of some singers to shatter a glass. The reason for this is that the note they sing happens to be the same as the natural vibrating frequency of the glass.

Now if we allow vibrations to go through our spine that are the same as the spine's natural vibrating frequency, it may not shatter, but it will have a weakening effect on the structures of the spine over a period of time. So someone who is driving for a living, or operating some form of machinery, may find that the vibration effect builds up over the years and weakens the spine. Is there any way you can reduce the amount of vibration that you experience?

What Can Go Wrong

Vibrations can also increase the amount of pain that you may already be feeling. For example, a milkman that we knew of, having learnt about the effects of vibration, discovered that if he sat on a 4in (100mm) foam cushion when driving his milk float, which did not have any shock absorbers, his pain virtually disappeared.

JERKY MOVEMENTS

Our bodies have built-in protective reflexes which come into play if we try to do something that is likely to cause us harm. However, if we make a sudden, jerky movement, these reflexes do not have a chance to work and damage may occur. It is, therefore, important that all our movements should always be smooth and well co-ordinated.

REFERRED PAIN

Pain is not always felt only in the back. It is quite possible that pain may be experienced in a different place from where it actually originates. For example, you may feel a pain in the calf of your leg, or even just a numb big toe, but that pain or sensation is actually coming from the spine. This is known as referred pain, as the pain is generated in one part of the body and referred to another, where it is felt.

Let us think about why and how this happens. You can tear a disc and not know that you have damaged it. Any one of us could be walking around with a torn disc and be totally unaware of it because, unlike a cut hand, which is decidedly painful, the disc does not have any nerve endings that 'feel' pain. It is not until a part of that torn disc moves and starts pressing on something which does have nerve endings, that you feel any pain.

Generally speaking, if the torn disc presses on the liga-

What Can Go Wrong

ments in your back, you get back pain; and if it presses on a nerve you get referred pain to the area served by that nerve.

The nerves coming out from the spinal cord pass through little gaps formed at either side of the spine where each two vertebrae join together. The nerves that come out in the neck region go down into your arms. Those that come out of the lower back go into your legs, and the nerves coming out of the 'middle' (the thoracic spine) supply the trunk and the organs inside.

Depending which nerve is being pressed upon, you will feel pain in an area supplied by that nerve. If the nerves in the neck are pressed, you feel pain down the arm. Nerves in the lower back give rise to pain down the leg, commonly known as 'sciatica'. Nerves in the thoracic spine can create pains that may feel like a heart problem or a gall-bladder problem.

For those of you who have experienced referred pain, you will probably know that there are also other symptoms that will be felt. You may have a feeling like tingling, numbness, burning, rushing water, a tight band around the limb; a whole range of sensations, just because the nerves are being irritated by a back pain problem.

When the torn piece of disc moves back into its normal position, the pain will go away. However, unlike a cut hand, which will bleed, form a scab and heal up, discs do not have a blood supply, so they can never heal up completely. It is quite likely to shift out of position again in the future, particularly if you continue with stooping, twisting, vibrations or jerky movements. This does unfortunately mean that once you have developed a disc problem, you will have it for life.

But, if you look after your back, think about what you are doing and avoid the things that have probably contributed to your problem, you may be able to go through life with the minimum of pain and discomfort.

The little facet joints in your back can also produce

referred pain. If you sprain or tear the facet joints, they will swell up, just as a sprained ankle swells. As the nerves run right over the little facet joints, where they leave the spinal cord, it does not require much swelling before there is pressure on the nerve, and referred pain is generated.

BACK PAIN IN WOMEN

During pregnancy, the body releases hormones quite early on to slacken the ligaments in the pelvis and lumbar spine. This allows more room for the baby and enables the birth to be more easily achieved. This is very positive of course, but, unfortunately, all the time that these ligaments are slack, the joints are more able to wobble to some extent, and they can then be overstretched and damaged very easily. It is worthwhile remembering that these hormones continue to be released for about four months after the baby has been born. At this time, with a new baby and perhaps buckets of nappies to lift, your back is very vulnerable. Many women have found that this was the time when their back pain problems first started.

These hormonal changes also occur, to a lesser degree, within the monthly menstrual cycle. If you are someone who does experience increased aching at a particular time of the month, then do take this as a warning sign. Your ligaments can be slackened by the action of your hormones, and you will be at increased risk of causing some damage.

By now, you can probably begin to understand why it can be so difficult to make a precise diagnosis as to what is wrong with your back, or what is actually causing your particular back pain. There are so many different structures that may be damaged, in a relatively small area, which can all give rise to similar signs and symptoms. It is for this very reason that back pain can be difficult to treat and does not necessarily respond to a standard treatment.

4
Reducing the Stress

We now know that most back pain is created by the stresses we place on the structures within our backs. In order to combat these stresses we must look at the way we move and position our bodies during our everyday lives. The postures that we have adopted in our civilised way of life are not always what is best for our bodies, and in particular, our backs.

SITTING

Of the three basic positions of sitting, standing and lying, we know that sitting produces most pressure or stress on the spine. Bearing this in mind, there are three important things to remember when you are sitting down. First, it is important to ensure your lower back is always comfortably supported and that there is no room for daylight to pass between your back and the back of the chair. There are many ways of achieving this. You could use a hot water bottle (not too hot), or a cushion, or rolled-up towel, for example.

Secondly, if you sit in your seat bolt upright, with a ninety degree angle at your hips, then there will be considerably more stress on the spine than if you are able to open out the angle to more than ninety degrees.

Thirdly, do make sure that there is at least a little bit of bend at your knees. If you sit with your legs out completely straight, you will be pulling on your hamstring muscles at the back of your thighs, which then pull your lower back into a stooped posture.

If you are sitting down and involved in some form of

activity, such as reading, sewing, knitting or doing a crossword, try to make sure that you rest your elbows on the arms of the chair. By doing this you will find that a great deal of tension will be removed from the muscles of the upper arm and neck, which occurs whenever you hold anything in your hands.

DESK WORK AND TYPING

Most modern-day desks have a flat, horizontal surface and to be able to work at this surface, the spine is encouraged to stoop. The solution to this is to have a work surface which is able to slope. This sloping surface allows us to sit with the spine in a natural, more upright posture. A draughtsman's table is an ideal example of this. A sloping surface can be made from various materials, and there are also commercial ones available.

An ergonomically-designed chair has a seat that is either sloped forward, or is able to slope forward with the user. Sitting on a chair with a forward-sloping seat has two benefits; first, the angle at your hip joints opens up to more than ninety degrees, which we have already discussed as being beneficial. Secondly, the pelvis is tilted forward, which allows your spine to achieve its natural 'S' shaped curve. This improved sitting posture reduces pressure on the spine quite considerably, which resumes the posture it normally adopts when standing. It is for these reasons that many people who are unable to sit in a conventional chair, because of the pain, are often able to sit and work on an ergonomically-designed chair.

An economical way of achieving a sloped seating surface, is simply to place a wedge-shaped piece of foam on to the flat seat of a conventional chair.

However you sit, if you are leaning forward, the pressure on the spine increases, but if you are writing for example, you

Reducing the Stress

are often leaning on the desk with your arms. In doing this a certain amount of the weight of your trunk is taken by your arms and not by your spine, thus reducing the amount of pressure exerted on the spinal structures. When you are sitting down, it is always worth remembering that the particular activity you are involved in can make the pressure on the spine either increase or decrease in the same way as if you were standing. Whenever you are doing anything in front of you, if you can lean on the working surface with your trunk or arms, this can help to reduce the pressure on your back.

In schools of the past, there was a row of sloping desks, with a row of sloping forms to sit on. For some inexplicable reason we decided to take a step backwards in evolution and flatten out both our writing surface and seating! How many children get into trouble at school nowadays because they tilt their chair forward on the front two legs? Not a good idea from a safety point of view, but they are only trying to put their back into a natural shape when doing desk work. No one teaches them to do it, this is the body trying naturally to protect itself.

If you are copy-typing, try to make sure that the work you are copying is fixed in front of you, rather than to one side. One of the worst places for the work you are copying is on the desk at the side of the typewriter, as this causes the neck to remain permanently stooped and twisted as you read the work. There are several commercial types of stand available, or it may be quite adequate to pin or stick the work to the wall in front of you, using a reusable adhesive such as BluTac.

With all desk work it is important that the desk surface is at a comfortable height for you. If it isn't, then try to get it altered otherwise you will develop unnecessary aches and pains.

Reducing the Stress

THE 'RULES' OF HANDLING

If we study the back and what causes the majority of back pain to arise, we can formulate what can be called the 'rules' of handling. We call them 'rules', but they can really only be guidelines as there are sure to be many occasions when, for one reason or another, you will not be able to apply all of the 'rules'. There are six basic 'rules', which involve checking your body posture to ensure that you are in the best possible position, or shape, for carrying out any particular task. If you can obey some of them and thereby get yourself into the best possible position for a particular situation, you can reduce the risk of injuring yourself or aggravating your present condition.

1 Back straight

Perhaps the longest-standing rule of handling and lifting is to keep your back straight. By talking about keeping the back straight, we mean try to keep your spine in its correct 'S' shaped curve. Remember that straightening out the natural curves will actually weaken the spine. Avoid the stooped posture (*see* Fig 5) and use your legs to squat down.

There will be many occasions when you can't use a squatting posture; perhaps because you have painful knees, or because of the poor design of equipment. In situations such as these you can maintain a fairly good posture by sticking your bottom out and pivoting at the hip joints. This may not look very elegant, and at first you will probably feel a bit self-conscious of this new way of bending, but remember that it is good for your back. Although you are leaning forwards, because you are pivoting at the hip joints, your back is inclined forward in an 'S' shape rather than being stooped. In some circumstances it may well be more convenient to pivot at one hip joint, allowing the other leg to extend out behind you to act as a counterbalance.

Reducing the Stress

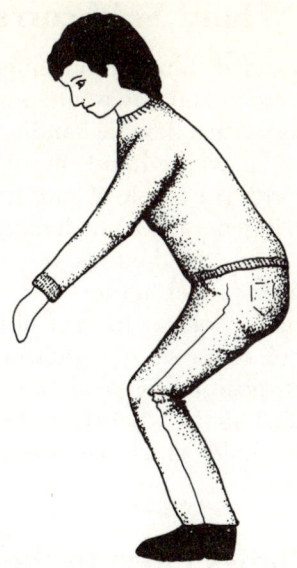

Fig 6   Ape-style lifting.

Keeping your back straight also includes trying to avoid twisting your back. Think of the 'carrot' effect discussed earlier in Chapter 3. If you have to turn around then move your feet, either by taking small steps or pivoting on your heels and toes.

If you are squatting to lift something, particularly if it is on the heavy side, then the full squat is not recommended. You can put yourself into a far stronger position to lift if you combine squatting with sticking your bottom out (*see* Fig 6).

Whenever you use the squat position your thigh muscles, which are big and strong, do the work of lifting. If you lift from a stooped position you are using the small muscles of the back to do all the work and these are much more easily injured. Using the thigh muscles is also less tiring, and although your leg muscles may ache a little to begin with, this will soon stop as they strengthen up with use.

Reducing the Stress

2   Hand hold correct

Most of us have carried things in our fingertips and felt the strain right up our arm and down into our backs. If you are carrying something with a flexible handle, like a carrier bag, then try putting your whole hand through the handle and grasping the bag with the whole of your hand instead of just your fingers. This is generally a much more comfortable and relaxed grip, and as an added bonus, very often what you are carrying will appear to feel lighter.

If you are going to hold or lift any object, start off with your hand in a hook shape so that you can mould your hand around the object, positioning your hand into the shape of the object. Again, using the whole hand to grip gives a much more relaxed hand hold which will lessen the stress felt in your arm and spine.

3   Elbows close to the body

Always try to keep your elbows tucked in close to the sides of your body. By doing this you are more likely to keep the object within your base, and you are more able to stabilise the load you are handling against your body. There should be no room for daylight to pass between your body and whatever you are carrying or lifting. By keeping the load against you, some of the weight is transmitted through your body rather than being taken by your arms. This will make the task of lifting a lot easier for you.

4   Foot position stable

Where you place your feet is very important. When you are standing up with your feet comfortably apart, you feel stable. If you lean your body forward, without moving your feet, then you become unstable, even without lifting anything. In order that the minimum stress is put on your back, you must try to keep your centre of gravity within your base, that is between your feet. There will be many situations where either one or both of your knees can be used effectively as 'feet'. Every time you move, your centre of gravity moves, and in order to remain stable you have to alter your foot position. This will help you to avoid stooping and twisting, so, whenever you move, move your feet. When you are lifting anything remember to get the load as close as possible.

5 Head up – chin in

When you are getting ready to lift, lift up your head. This will help to straighten the whole of your spine. Try this now; lift your head up into a natural upright position and feel how the rest of your spine straightens automatically. Gently tucking in your chin helps to protect your neck. You may have your head and neck stooped and twisted, in order to see what you are doing, as you prepare to lift something. When you are ready to lift, lift your head into its natural posture, gently tucking in your chin to reduce the risk of injuring your neck through the stress placed on it by your posture.

6 Body weight

You don't necessarily have to be big and strong to handle relatively heavy and awkward loads. If you have a good technique, then your own body weight will do a lot of the work for you.

Once you begin to handle or lift anything, try to make it a continuous movement ensuring that you lift, move, and put the load down in a smooth and co-ordinated way, without any jerky movements. Use your body's momentum to propel you forward as this reduces the amount of energy that you have to use. Do not confuse the use of momentum with running. Running, whilst handling or lifting, inevitably increases the risk of accidents and injury occurring as the movement cannot be smooth and becomes jerky. Body weight can also be used effectively to push and pull loads instead of carrying them.

The six 'rules' are worth remembering and by quickly running through them in your mind whenever you handle anything, you will almost certainly alter your body shape or position in some way. This will reduce the risk of injury.

WHAT CLOTHES TO WEAR

Whenever you are going to be involved in handling or lifting things, think about the clothes you are wearing at the time. It is quite possible that they can make life easy for you, but it's equally likely that they can make life a lot more difficult, if not actually hazardous. Ideally you need clothes that are loose and comfortable, that will allow you to move easily, and enable you to get into the correct position for lifting. Watch out for such things as watches, rings, brooches, badges, screwdrivers or pens sticking out of pockets which can all catch on what you are handling, and cause you to make a sudden jerky movement. This, if you remember, is one of the four things that you should try to avoid. The other three are stooping, twisting and vibrations.

Shoes should have a supporting, flat, non-slip sole, be well-fitting and cover the whole of your foot. For anyone dealing with heavy objects protective steel toe caps are an obvious recommendation, in fact, a must.

Females have two main problems with traditional clothing; shoes and skirts. If you are handling and lifting things, high heels and sling-backs, or shoes with no backs at all, can potentially be very dangerous. With this type of footwear your heel could very easily slip off the shoe and cause injury to the ankle. Even a small heel reduces the stability of your base, which, as previously discussed, is not helpful when handling things. We have known patients who have complained of quite severe back pain to be 'cured' just by wearing lower heels. When you wear high heels, particularly for long periods of time, you are forced to stand forward on your toes. Because your weight is being thrown forward you automatically lean backwards to compensate (remember that we always try to keep our centre of gravity within our base). This leaning results in an increase in the curve in your lower back, which 'crunches' the little facet joints together. So, walking around in your high heels, you are literally grinding the bones together. It's really not surprising that people with high heels often develop backache.

If you have to handle something that is, for example, slippery or sharp, then consider wearing a pair of gloves. Gloves of the right size and made of a suitable material may well enable you to gain a much better grip. Be aware that some gloves are unsuitable for handling items of certain other materials. For example, if you're holding something wet with smooth plastic gloves, there could be more chance of your hands slipping than if you were to use your bare hands. There may also be other factors to consider, such as is the material corrosive?

ASSESSING THE LOAD

Always assess the weight of anything before you attempt to move it. This can be achieved by either tilting it gently from side to side, or by using a trial lift. To assess the weight of a large item, get yourself into position as if you are ready to lift, but instead of lifting the object just take the strain, then relax your effort and decide whether you are going to be able to move it yourself, or whether you need some help.

Despite any tables or statistics that may be quoted, only you know how much you can lift. Some days you will find that you feel capable of handling more than on other days.

Reducing the Stress

We all have our off days when we are unable to do the things that we know we can normally do. The important thing to remember is that if you don't feel that you can manage to lift something comfortably, then don't lift it! Get some help, either in the form of other people to assist you, or perhaps some kind of mechanical gadget. A mechanical gadget can be anything, from something as sophisticated as a fork-lift truck to something as simple as an old rug which can be used to pull things along on.

Another reason for assessing the weight before handling anything is that quite a few people can develop back problems as a result of picking up very light things. A common example is the empty dustbin. People very often assume that a dustbin will be full and heavy and lift it, using effort far in excess of that required, so that the dustbin comes up with such a sudden jerk that their back is damaged. In this case it is not the weight of the item that has caused the damage, it is the jerky movement.

Avoid lifting anything without considering whether there is another way that the item can be shifted. Can you use some form of mechanical gadget? Can you push it with your foot? Can you lean against it and push it with your body weight? Use your imagination and think carefully before you lift it. However, be careful if you are going to pull anything one handed, as it is very easy to twist your spine whilst it is loaded, putting a heavy stress on your back.

Assessing the load, however small or large it may be, will become easier as you practice it. Just being aware that the load may not be as secure as it appears, nor the weight that it looks, is enough to warrant an assessment for your own sake.

TEAMWORK

When you have to handle objects with the assistance of one or more people, there are advantages and disadvantages to

Reducing the Stress

be aware of. The major advantage is that by sharing the task, the amount of load taken by each individual member of the team will be greatly reduced. However, there is also one major disadvantage which is the risk of something going wrong, and an injury to your back occurring can be greatly increased. It is therefore very important to act together as a well co-ordinated team when handling anything with other people. One person should act as the co-ordinator, giving commands and ensuring that everybody moves together at the right time in a smooth and co-ordinated way. Before actually committing themselves to the lift, everyone should know exactly how the object is going to be picked up, what route is going to be taken, and what is going to happen to it when you get to the other end. If at any time a member of the team needs to stop, perhaps because they feel that they are losing their grip, then stop immediately. Put the object down in a co-ordinated way, safely, for everyone. Don't be tempted to say 'hold on, we're nearly there' because if they lose their grip completely, the extra weight will be forced on to the other members of the team in a jerky fashion which will quite likely cause injury to one, if not more, of the people involved.

Ideally, it is useful to use people of a similar height to work together in a team. If this is possible the weight of the object being carried will be evenly shared amongst the lifters. When two people of unequal height lift a table, and both take hold of the table at the same height and both stand up straight, the shorter person is going to bear all the weight. However, the weight can be balanced more evenly between the two, providing they are prepared to work together as a team. This can be achieved in one of two ways. First, the shorter person may be able to hold the table lower down. In this way the table is then level when they both stand upright. Secondly, the taller person should bend his knees until he is roughly the same height as his partner, remembering not to stoop. There may be occasions when the shorter person holds the object lower and the taller person also needs to bend his knees. Always remember that working together as a team and looking after each other will make the handling task a lot safer, and certainly a lot easier.

SHOPPING

Try not to go shopping on your own. You will find that a helpmate makes all the difference. If you are out shopping for a few individual items, take two bags with you (carrier bags fold up very small and can be used more than once). In this way you can carry one in each hand and balance out the load. Remember that you can carry a greater load in more comfort this way, rather than carrying the whole load in one hand.

If your shopping expedition takes you into the supermarkets, always take a trolley rather than a basket, even if you only need a few things. Steering the infamous supermarket trolley may be a problem; try to find a good one before entering the store.

Some of the following suggestions may be of assistance if you've not already tried some of them. Have a go with them and see if they make life any easier for you. When there are two of you, having one person to guide the front end of the trolley is helpful. On your own you may find it easier pushing it sideways on, or if it is one that tends to want to run to one side, try pushing it by the handle, aiming towards the opposite shelves. The trolley very often ends up travelling easily up the aisle. Pulling the trolley is another alternative, but this is not always appropriate in a busy store, and if you are pulling it you can normally only do it with one hand, so be very careful that you do not let your spine twist while you are doing it.

When you are putting things into the trolley, drop them in if you can. If not, try standing at the sides or lowest end of the trolley. Put a hand on the opposite side of the trolley to

Reducing the Stress

support the weight of your trunk and stabilise the trolley. Then lean forward, pivoting at your hip joints and keeping your spine in a straight, natural posture as you place the item in with your other hand. If there is no one behind you, it is possible to achieve an even better position by allowing one leg to stretch out behind as you pivot on the other hip joint. This leg then acts as a counterbalance. Raising the base of the trolley can be achieved if you don't need to fill it, by placing an upturned basket or box in the bottom. This is worth trying, as you then don't have so far to reach down when loading and unloading the trolley.

When you get to the check-out, bring the trolley through the aisle after you, with the handle away from you. In this position it can be unloaded using the same technique described above; one hand on the trolley, pivoting at the hip joint, with one leg acting as counterbalance, using your other hand to unload the items. Be careful at this point not to twist as you place the goods on the check-out. If you have a heavy item that requires both hands to lift it out, stand at the corner of the trolley and bend your knees. This will enable you to keep the load as close to you as possible without stooping forward.

Don't be tempted to use the large shopping trolley bags available to fit into the shopping trolley. To lift one of these, when full, or even partly full, can only be achieved by leaning forward and using your back to try and lift it out, even if there are two of you. Generally, you are better off using smaller baskets, boxes or carrier bags.

When you go to put the shopping into your car, put the trolley into a suitable position before transferring the load, to avoid any unnecessary stooping or twisting. You will also find that it is often best to put things into the boot rather than inside the car.

Trying to put things into and get things out of a car boot can be awkward. To achieve it whilst maintaining a good posture can be quite a problem. Estate cars and hatchbacks

Reducing the Stress

can be easier as you are able to place the load on the rim, lean against it and use body weight to just push it into the car.

Getting things in and out of a car boot is probably best achieved by doing it in two or three stages:

(1) Lift the load and place it on the rim of the boot.
(2) If you have something such as an upturned sturdy box acting as a platform inside the boot, slide the load from the rim of the boot on to the platform using your body weight.
(3) Gently guide the load on to the floor of the boot from the platform.

Standing at the corner of the boot will also enable you to achieve a better position. When you stand at the back of the car, you cannot bend your knees, and you are then likely to stoop over into the boot. By positioning yourself at the corner, you are able to bend your knees with the corner of the car between your legs, allowing you to get the load within your base.

With many more bulky loads, such as a sack of potatoes or a bag of cement, a very useful technique is to put one foot in the boot of the car. In this way you are able to get much closer to the load and to lift it on to the rim again, keeping the weight within your base. With the load safely balanced on the rim of the boot, alter your foot position, and lift the load off the car. Notice that with all these suggestions the task has been broken down into several stages allowing you to alter your position to a more stable one for the next stage.

If you have an estate car or hatchback, an old rug on the floor will make it easier to push the load in, and when you are unloading, you can pull the rug towards you, bringing the load to the edge of the car for you to lift it off. This method often helps you to avoid having to clamber into the car and try to lift the load out when you are forced into an awkward and poor posture.

Reducing the Stress

WASHING

Washing clothes can be quite a chore for the back pain sufferer, as it can involve quite heavy and awkward loads. First of all, think about where you actually do the washing. Is it easy to get at? Is it at the best height for you to be able to handle the washing which increases its weight quite dramatically when it is wet? If you are using a washing machine and tumble dryer, are they easy to load? Front loaders are often in base units under a work top, but this does make it hard work to load and unload the washing. Consider whether it may be more convenient for the main user if the machine could be fitted into a housing similar to that of a split-level cooker. With a suitable work surface or table close by, there need be no bending involved in either loading or unloading the washing. When planning a utility room or kitchen spend time giving this very serious thought.

With the washing done, don't try to lift the whole load into a big linen basket all in one go. When hanging out the washing use smaller baskets or perhaps a bowl, so that you carry a lighter load. This may mean making more than one trip to the washing line, but it will be better for your back in the long run. Research has shown that it is better to make several journeys carrying a lighter load, than to make one journey carrying the whole lot. Make sure that your washing line can be lowered to a height that you are able to reach without having to stretch. Remember that when you stretch up there is a tendency to lean back, increasing the curve in your back and causing the facet joints to crunch together. This will lead to additional aches and pains. When collecting in the washing always remember that the items that you are taking off the line may be very small and light, but the way that you stand, and the way that you actually handle this small, insignificant item, may just be the cause of a painful back problem. This is particularly important to remember when you are in a hurry to get the dry washing in because of

Reducing the Stress

the rain. In addition to your posture whilst collecting the washing, there is the added hazard of slipping on a wet surface or tripping over something which may be obscured by the load you are carrying.

IRONING

Don't put off the ironing until you have a big pile of it to do. A great deal of ironing will make anyone liable to get backache. On occasions when there is a lot of ironing to be done, just iron a few things, go away and do something else for a while, then come back and iron a few more items, and do something else again. This will help to ease the burden, because even if you like ironing, you are handling a relatively heavy piece of equipment and moving it backwards and forwards in a way that can generate fatigue. Make sure that you have adjusted the height of the ironing board so that it is right for you, depending on whether you prefer to stand or sit, so that you are able to keep your back in its natural shape. If you sit down to iron, be sure that you have a suitable support in the small of your back (it need only be something like a small towel), and that you can open out the angle of the hips and lean back in the chair as you are ironing.

If you stand up to do your ironing and find that your back aches, try standing with one foot up on a small step; two telephone directories are often at just about the right height. Always position yourself as close to the board as possible to avoid having to stoop. Some people have found that if they stand up and perch themselves on the edge of a table, they can do their ironing in comfort. Obviously if you are going to lean back against something like a table you need to ensure that it won't move whilst you are working.

When there are a lot of creases to be ironed out, it is often better to stand sideways on to the board, so that you can transfer your body weight from your backward foot to your forward foot to avoid twisting your spine. By getting too engrossed in the creases, there is a tendency to begin to stoop lower and lower as you iron. Be aware of your posture and correct it, if you feel it is becoming worse. Be careful that you don't twist the spine as you pick up items from one pile and, having ironed them, place them on the completed pile. Use your feet and move your base.

WORKTOPS AND WORKBENCHES

Many people develop back ache when they are standing and working at a work surface, because to be able to reach their work and see what they are doing, their back tends to get into a slightly stooped posture. To combat this you could try putting one foot up on to some kind of small step. By just slightly altering the mechanics of the body, this will very often take away that troublesome ache.

When standing at the kitchen sink, try opening the cupboard door and putting your foot on the base shelf. If the washing-up bowl is low, place an upturned bowl under the one you are using. When in a workshop or shed, a tin can, brick, lump of wood etc. will suffice, if the workbench doesn't already have a suitable rung across the front.

Look at the height of the working surface to see if it is comfortable for you to work at. If the surface is too high for you then try using a platform to stand on. If the surface is too low, causing you to stoop, then it may be worth building or buying a false platform that you are able to place on the surface if you are going to be working there for more than about ten minutes.

Reducing the Stress

WORKING AT FLOOR LEVEL

Whenever you have to work down at floor level, such as when cleaning or laying floor coverings, the best approach is to get down on 'all fours', using knee-pads if necessary. In this way the weight of your trunk is supported on your hands and knees, and your spine is 'slung' straight between them. This prevents the strain that would be put on your spine by kneeling or squatting on the floor and stooping forward or twisting to the side to reach whatever you are working on. By using the 'all fours' position, your neck is also better protected as it is in line with your trunk and you do not have to stoop or twist to the side to see what you are doing. If it's possible, the easy answer with cleaning is to use a long-handled mop and stand up.

VACUUMING AND SWEEPING

Whilst you are using a broom or long-handled cleaner, try to keep your head up and your chin in. It is very easy to become so engrossed in what you are cleaning that you begin to allow your spine to stoop. Make good use of your body weight, always moving your feet as you clean. Avoid the temptation to twist your spine but use your feet instead to turn the whole body round. Apply the six 'rules'.

With a cylinder cleaner, check the length of the rigid pipe to see if you can comfortably move it around without having to bend forward. It may be worth trying to get an extension piece of tubing to allow yourself to stand in a more upright posture. If you are thinking of buying a new cleaner, or any piece of equipment for that matter, do think carefully about how it will affect you and your back. When possible, try it out before you buy it. Some cleaners can be very heavy or difficult to handle, putting unnecessary strain on your back.

Vacuuming the stairs can be a problem, whichever type of

cleaner you use. Always stand on a stair lower than the ones you're cleaning. It may be worthwhile investing in a small rechargeable cleaner for areas like the stairs. Some people who suffer with back pain find it far more comfortable to push the vacuum cleaner round the house on their hands and knees.

DECORATING AND CLEANING

Whenever you are doing this sort of work, the difficulty is to avoid looking up too high or leaning backwards for any length of time; for example, when painting a ceiling, cleaning windows, hanging curtains etc. Remember the effect that this position has on the facet joints of the back and neck. Although you may only feel slight discomfort at the time, it can cause quite severe pain that will not become apparent until the following day. There are many tools available on the market today which can make life considerably easier for jobs that do require us to reach up to them. Long-handled mops or dusters are available for cleaning, and most specialist decorating stores sell decorating rollers which are suitable for use with an extension handle. By using these long-handled tools, you do not have to look directly above you, but are able to work more ahead of yourself, keeping your head and neck in a more natural position. There are occasions where the situation you are working in dictates that you must work directly above you. With this situation, repeatedly bring your head down to a natural position for a few seconds.

WORKING ON THE CAR

Working under the bonnet of a car is one situation where you are forced to lean forward, so remember to stick your bottom out and pivot at the hips! Very often in this situation you are able to lean on your arms, or elbows, so that your arms are supporting the weight of your trunk, not the muscles of your back. You can experience these two different positions by standing in front of a table. Just become aware of the muscles in your back and feel how much they are working. Now put your hands on the edge of the table, and lean the weight of your body on them. As you do this you should immediately feel the muscles in your back relaxing.

Whilst under the bonnet of a car, if you have to work even lower in the engine bay, then rest your chest across the top, allowing the car to support the entire weight of your trunk, leaving both hands free to work. Some form of protection, such as a folded piece of carpet, can make this more comfortable for you to lean on. Placing one knee on the bumper can often get you into a more comfortable position. Always try to support the weight of your trunk on your arms or hands whenever you're doing anything in front of you, whether you are standing or sitting. This will reduce the amount of compression force on the spine which will occur if your back muscles have to do all the work.

Don't stay working in this sort of position for too long, otherwise you may well get stuck, and be unable to straighten up! Every now and then just straighten up carefully and have a short break before you return to your work.

WORKING AT LOW LEVELS

Another awkward working position is at a low level, when you may need to work on your knees or in a squatting position. In this position avoid stooping your neck; keep your head up and chin in and let your eyes do the looking down. Whenever it's possible, always work directly in front of you. If you work to one side, you will twist your spine and it will not be very long before you begin to feel discomfort in your back. Also, if you have to carry out something forceful whilst you are twisted to one side, such as screwdriving, you could quite easily 'tweak' something, as the muscles pull hard on a distorted spine.

BABIES AND CHILDREN

Handling and lifting people is not straightforward and has, indeed, been the subject of training courses and books in its own right. This is due to the flexibility and unpredictability of the human being. Children, particularly younger children and babies, create added problems. Modern baby furniture and nursery equipment tends to be designed very much with the safety of the baby in mind. Little ergonomic thought appears to go to the parents who have the task of handling both the child and the equipment. The mother has the additional problem, as mentioned earlier, that for approximately four months after the baby is born, her ligaments are still vulnerable through slackness created by hormonal activity.

When handling youngsters there is a considerable amount of carrying to do. The amount of time spent in a poor posture can increase dramatically if you are not extra careful.

A nursing mother, feeding her baby either by breast or bottle, will often have a tendency to look at the baby. This involves a stoop and twist of the neck, and it is not therefore recommended. Some mothers like to watch the baby, as they are worried that it may suffocate on the breast. In this context there is nothing to worry about as the baby's nose is shaped in such a way as to prevent this happening. Also the active suckling baby is normally quite capable of moving itself if it cannot breathe adequately.

When carrying a small child or baby be aware that there is a tendency to lean backwards to compensate for the load. Remember that by leaning backwards you will place in-

Reducing the Stress

creased stress on to your facet joints, so it is best to try and keep yourself as upright as you can.

If you are going to be holding a baby for any length of time while standing up, you may find it helpful if you are able to lean against a wall or perch on something like the edge of a table. Many people find a baby carrier useful for carrying a baby for any distance, but do check on your posture, perhaps by using a mirror, before using one of these for any length of time. It is also worth remembering that many baby slings and carriers are designed to be worn on your back. These make it easier for you to keep a good posture, but you may need assistance putting them on and taking them off.

With slightly bigger children, many parents tend to carry them with the child sitting astride one hip. This enables the weight of the child to be transferred down through the pelvis to the leg, avoiding the spine completely. However, there can be a tendency when carrying a child on one hip to shift the spine sideways in order to balance it. Obviously this is not a good posture to adopt, so again, try to keep yourself and your spine as upright as possible.

Great benefit can be gained if you are able to rest for short periods between activities as well, preferably by lying down in the psoas position (*see* Fig 8). Remember to keep to the six 'rules' as closely as you can, bearing in mind the difficulties that are often experienced with equipment designed for the baby, but not designed for you.

With many of the cots, prams, baby bouncers and commercial changing areas generally available today, it is very often not possible to get into a good, stable position. It is in this situation that you may find the best alternative position is to pivot forward at the hips, keeping your back straight, perhaps using one leg as a counterbalance. It would be easy, when faced with this situation, to give in to the old habit of stooping, because you are in a hurry.

When you are making the cot up, rest one hand on the opposite side of the cot, as you lean forward, in order to

Reducing the Stress

support the weight of your trunk through your arm and not your back. Remember also, that your knees can make very good feet! When you are using the baby bouncer, for example, rather than standing and bending forward, you may find it easier to kneel by the side of it and, if necessary bend forward at the hips.

Pushing a pram or pushchair can easily encourage you to stoop if you are not careful about maintaining your posture. It is worth checking that the handle is at a comfortable height for the main user. For a good position your elbows should be slightly bent. You can make good use of your body weight while pushing prams, especially when starting off and also when going up or down steps or kerbs. To use your body weight when you are going up a step, place one foot on the footrest, if the pram has one, then stand up on your toes. Keeping your arms straight, come down off your toes, and the front wheels of the pram will lift.

When designing a nursery for the baby, try to design it ergonomically, bearing in mind that the adult involved with the care of the infant will spend plenty of time in there undertaking essential activities on a regular basis. The changing area, for instance, should be a raised area that is around about the hip height of the main user. In some houses, where there is a boxed area over the stairwell in one of the bedrooms, this can be quite easy to achieve. The changing mat can be supported at hip height and the area is protected on other sides by walls. If this is not possible, then it is better for you to change the baby on a table, or kneel by the side of a bed, chair or sofa. Never leave any child unattended on a raised surface.

Bathing the baby can pose quite a problem. When you use a baby bath, try to arrange for it to be as close as possible to the water supply. This will help you to avoid having to carry the bath whilst it is full of water. This on its own is not an easy task, as the water makes the load you are carrying very unstable. One solution that has proved to be ideal for some

Reducing the Stress

parents, is to place the baby bath into the family bath, preferably on a stable stand of some kind. With the baby bath safely supported at a convenient height, you will not have to bend over as much when using it. You will also be able to fill the baby bath using a shower attachment fixed to the bath taps. With a baby that is not too much of a 'wriggler', a folded towel on the toilet seat can make a convenient place to undress it. Wherever the baby bath is, you will have to lean forward slightly to put the baby in. In this situation you are able to kneel down and use the side of the big bath to lean against as you place the baby into the baby bath, and then take it out.

Although there are many people using disposable nappies these days, a considerable number of people still prefer to use washable 'terry' nappies. When these have to be carried in buckets, it is far better to carry two, one in each hand, so that you are well balanced. Although you may be carrying a greater weight, it actually feels easier, and is less stressful on the spine than carrying one bucket, so consider purchasing two small buckets rather than one large one.

For people who prefer to use disposable nappies, a number of firms, in several countries, now offer a free delivery service, which means that you do not have to carry bulky packs from the shops. Having someone else to carry the packs of nappies for you often means buying in bulk. If you cannot afford to buy in bulk yourself, you may know of a friend or neighbour who will go halves to help you both out.

One particular difficulty with handling children is trying to lift them in or out of a car. For the safety of all occupants, all children should ride in the rear seats and be secured in either a child's safety seat or harness. Lifting children in or out should be carried out carefully and with thought. Allow yourself enough time before your departure to avoid having to rush. You really need to give yourself as much room as possible by opening the doors and moving the front seat forward as far as it will go.

If there are two adults, it may be easier for one of you to be inside the car and position yourself as best you can to receive the child from the person outside. However you manage it, you are working in a confined space with a limited headroom. Try to obey the six 'rules' as closely as you are able to under the circumstances. Be very aware that this is a particularly difficult situation, so do take care.

SPORTS

Returning to sports or any sudden, prolonged active work after a relatively sedentary way of living should be approached with caution. Even non-sufferers should be aware of any sudden return to increased activity. The first bout of gardening of the year, the first game of the season and moving furniture are all quite likely to give you backache if you do not prepare yourself properly first. Always ease yourself in gradually with just a small amount of activity at first. As you progress, gradually increase the amount you do until you are up to a full, comfortable level.

If you are intending to return to a sporting activity, or take up a new one, always take it easy to start with and see how your back responds to it. Listen to what your back is telling you; if it continues to ache or give you pain, then that particular activity is most probably doing you more harm than good. In general, it is advisable to have some professional coaching before taking up any sport. This will enable you to get the best out of the sport, while at the same time protecting your body.

The importance of warming up and winding down is easily neglected. Whatever the activity, you should always go through some form of warming-up routine before you start. If you are a sufferer of low back pain, then it is wise to include stretching exercises for the hamstrings and calf muscles in your warm up. At the end of your session, gently wind down, to allow your body to return to its resting state naturally.

Swimming

Swimming is one of two sports that are generally recommended for back pain sufferers. In water you are only about a quarter of your normal body weight and so the pressure effects on the spine are greatly reduced. You can exercise more without putting too much stress on your spine.

There are, however, certain activities that should not be undertaken. Diving is best avoided, as this causes quite a severe jarring force on the spine. Using the butterfly stroke is also best avoided because of the considerable amount of spinal movement that is involved. If your particular problem is neck pain, and you use the breast stroke, holding your head out of the water whilst swimming is also likely to increase your pain.

Apart from general swimming there are a number of very useful exercises that you can do in water specifically to help strengthen and mobilise your back (*see* Chapter 6 for a section on 'Hydrotherapy'). Some people do find the normal swimming temperature to be cold, even to the point that it increases their pain, or they are unable to exercise because their muscles are too cold. If this is the case, enquire around your local swimming pools to see if any hold 'mother and toddler' or 'disabled persons' sessions. Pools that do hold sessions for these groups normally raise the temperature of the water for them, and if you go in for the next public session afterwards, you will probably find that the water is much warmer than normal.

Cycling

The second sport generally recommended for back pain sufferers is cycling. However, do bear in mind the four movements that you should try to avoid (stooping, twisting, vibrations, sudden jerks). Low handlebars are preferable because less jarring stress from the road surface is transmitted to the spine than if sitting in the upright position. Although with low handlebars your spine appears to be in the stooped posture, the weight of your trunk is taken through your arms and not directly through your spine. Avoid cycling over rough ground, or use a static bike instead.

SPORTS TO AVOID

Due to limited space we cannot go into the reasons in detail, but there are five sports that are particularly not recommended for back pain sufferers: water skiing, weight lifting, rowing, football and rugby. In general, avoid contact sports, sports which subject the spine to large compression forces, and sports using studded boots – the feet cannot pivot, and the spine has to twist as the player changes direction.

OTHER SPORTS

Aerobics – Yoga – Dancing

Having reached this part of the book, by now you will know what sort of movements are best avoided. Always listen to what your body is trying to tell you, and don't try to be too ambitious. Never try to work through pain (unless a specific medical supervisor is advising it for a particular condition in a controlled environment). Generally speaking the following exercises in aerobics should be avoided:

(1) Standing with your feet apart and bending over to touch your right foot with your left hand, or vice versa. This will involve both a stoop and a twist.

(2) Standing with your feet apart and twisting round from side to side at your waist. People are sometimes encouraged to 'bounce' at the extreme of each twist, which increases the amount of stress put on the disc.

(3) Lying on the floor with your legs straight, and then raising both legs upwards, together. This exercise puts a dangerous leverage on the spine and particularly places excessive strain on the female abdominal muscles.

Many people find the relaxation part of yoga a benefit to them, but avoid any of the positions that put stresses on their backs. These do sometimes aggravate or cause back pain problems.

Whichever style of dancing you involve yourself with, think carefully about any postures you adopt. Avoid the actions that you know should not be included.

Horse-Riding

Keep a good upright posture in the saddle, ensuring you maintain your natural lumbar curve. You may find that it is beneficial for you to wear a corset while riding, for support. A western-style saddle is often used to assist with the posture.

Tennis – Squash

Racket sports can lead to forceful twisting of the spine if you do not develop a good technique. Avoid twisting the back too much, try instead to turn by using your legs more, pivoting on your feet and bending at the hips and knees.

Golf

When walking around the golf course try to keep to relatively smooth ground, and use a golf trolley. Pulling the golf trolley is better than trying to push it, but beware the temptation of

Reducing the Stress

pulling with a twist in the spine. When teeing off, try to avoid a large follow through, twisting the spine, especially if you suffer with thoracic backache. Golf appears to aggravate the middle part of the thoracic spine in particular.

Jogging

Jogging should be a gentle exercise that is neither walking nor running. Wear suitable shock-absorbing shoes or insoles, particularly if you normally experience pain when standing or walking. These may also help to reduce this pain. Good shock-absorbing insoles are becoming more and more widely available, and are worth considering for everyday use. As you jog, keep erect, as opposed to leaning forwards. Take short strides and avoid any jolting steps. You should be able to hold a conversation with someone if you are jogging; if you can't because you're out of breath, you are 'pounding the streets' or running, not jogging. Select a route that does not include too many hard surfaces or uneven surface work. Small jogging trampolines are popular with some people, who are able to exercise gently, on a soft, absorbing surface in the privacy of their own home.

MOTORING

Many people experience backache travelling in motor vehicles. Often this is due to the combined stresses of sitting and vibrations. In order to become more comfortable when travelling in any form of transport, there are many things that may be adjusted or tried out.

Starting at the top of the seat and working down, look first of all at the head-rest. This should really be called the head restraint, because its real purpose is to restrain your head if you are unfortunate enough to be involved in a collision. If the vehicle in which you are travelling is brought to a sudden

Reducing the Stress

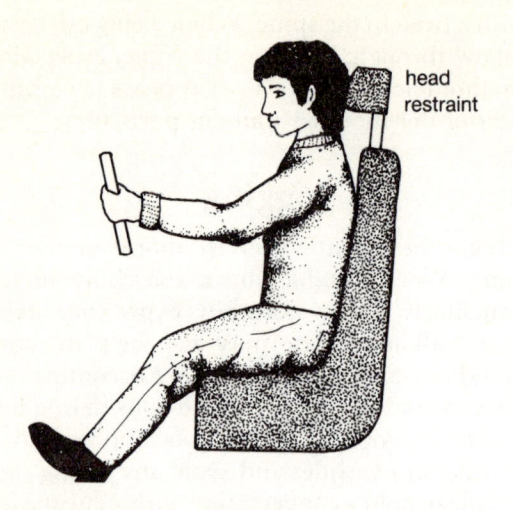

Fig 7 Driving position.

halt by a collision, your head, which is not restrained by any form of harness, is flung forwards, and then backwards, like a whip being lashed. This is where the term 'whiplash injury' comes from. A whiplash injury, although it primarily affects the neck, can also affect the lower parts of your back as the forces are transmitted through the spine from top to bottom.

If the head-rest on your seat is in the correct position, supporting your head and not your neck (*see* Fig 7), then the effects of a whiplash will be minimised, as your head will be restrained as it comes back and makes contact with the head-rest which absorbs the force. A head-rest in the wrong position, either too high or too low, can become a hazard, causing further injury, as the neck may be forced into an unnatural position. Should you not have a head-rest, it is worth investing in a good one, as, with seat belts now being worn, the whiplash effect is becoming more common.

The seat belt itself can create problems for some people as reaching for the inertia type involves twisting the spine.

Reducing the Stress

Good motor accessory shops sell a clip which allows you to pull through as much of the belt as you need, and then clip it off. In this way the belt will rest by the side of your seat when you are not using it, making it easier for you to reach.

Vehicle seats are now available with a wide range of adjustments. They can be reclined backwards and forwards, and the whole seat is adjustable backwards and forwards as well. We have been amazed at the number of people who, having suffered a lot of pain while driving, have gone home from our Backschools and been able to find a very comfortable driving position, just by trying different combinations of the above two adjustments.

You should have some support in your lower back. If the seat does not provide this, then use a small cushion, rolled-up towel, foam pad, or some other suitable support. A seat that has good support at the sides will create less stress and discomfort for the spine when going round corners.

For the person who suffers with back pain, but does a considerable amount of driving, a replacement car seat may be a worthwhile investment. There are a variety of replacement car seats available and it is therefore worthwhile looking around before you buy one. Some of the better ones can really cater for your individual requirements. Once you have purchased one of these, you can take it with you to your next car, provided you keep the old seat to put back into the car you are disposing of! Although these seats may be a little expensive, they can reduce a great deal of the stress on the spine, especially if the seat you have is damaged in any way, or has been moulded by use to the previous owner's shape.

GENERAL CARRYING

The way that we carry things can have a considerable effect on the development or aggravation of back pain. If we look at some of the countries around the world that still use head

Reducing the Stress

baskets and shoulder poles, we will see that they do not appear to suffer from the level of back pain that we in the western world do. Baskets and poles have been used throughout the world for centuries to carry things, and are excellent. The load is evenly balanced, and is brought as close to the centre of the body as possible. This avoids unnecessary leverage on the spine, which in turn causes unnecessary muscle work around the spine.

Today, we have forsaken these methods for alternative ways of carrying things. Whichever way you are using to carry anything, the more central you are able to get it, the better. Let's look at some of the ways you can achieve this. Carry things by cuddling them in front of you, or better still by using a rucksack. Because this is on your back it keeps you that much more upright, and helps to prevent you getting into a stooped posture. You can sometimes use your shoulder or hip to balance things on as you carry them. Supporting the load on your hip allows the weight of it to be transmitted directly from your pelvis to your leg, avoiding the spine completely. However, you must remember not to stick your hip out and thereby twist your spine; keep the posture of your back straight.

In situations where you have to carry things in your hands, always try to balance out and carry something in each hand. You will be able to safely handle a greater load if you balance out like this, with more comfort. Most of us can recall the aching we experience when we carry something one-handed.

Objects with handles are not always best carried by the handles. Before you pick something up by the handle and walk away with it stop for just a moment and think of what alternative ways could be used to carry it. You may well find that an easier method will come to mind. But, if you decide that you do have to carry something by its handle, keep your elbows tucked in and hold the handle just behind your hip. This position alters your centre of gravity slightly, helping to

Reducing the Stress

keep your spine straighter than if you were to carry it with your hand in front of your hip.

When using the handle to carry things by, remember to grip by using the whole of the hand, not just your fingertips. Most important of all, do you have to carry it at all? Can you pull it, push it, use your feet to move it, or perhaps use a mechanical gadget of some kind, a trolley or an old rug, for example, to avoid the stress on the spine that the weight of the object would generate.

Finally, when carrying anything, make sure that you are looking ahead of you and not down at the floor. Imagine that you have a book balanced on your head and you'll be in the best position to protect your back.

5
Coping with Back Pain

EASING AN ATTACK

Back pain can develop suddenly, or it can begin as a little ache which slowly develops into a severe pain. If you do develop any back pain or aching, or if you begin to experience more pain than is normal for you, stop whatever you are doing immediately. Either take a rest from activity, or do something else. Quite often a pain can be due to a particular posture that you are in, carrying out a particular activity. By changing what you are involved in, your posture will be altered and the pain may well ease off. Never think to yourself 'I'll just finish this', because pain is a warning signal, and working through it will make it worse, possibly causing more damage. You may not feel it at the time, but you will almost certainly suffer later. Remember to do what your back is trying to tell you.

If you decide to opt for a rest, one of the most useful positions is the psoas position (*see* Fig 8). (*See* also in Chapter 6, 'Rest'.) Try to use the psoas position as often as possible

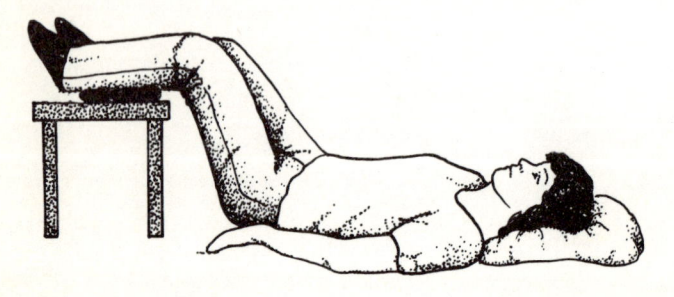

Fig 8   The psoas position.

when resting. You can use it in preference to sitting. Some people who use the psoas position enjoy watching television from this position and have even found it more comfortable than the armchair. Try to spend at least ten minutes at some time during your day in the psoas position. In this position you will be allowing the majority of the squashy, watery middle, which has been pushed out of the disc through pressure, to be taken back in again, allowing the disc to be more efficient.

WHAT BED SHOULD I HAVE?

The answer to this question is to choose a bed that suits you as an individual. Unfortunately, no specific type of bed can be recommended for all back pain sufferers. So often we have heard that if you have a problem with back pain, you are told to get a firmer bed. Sometimes this is true, but by no means is it always the case. The experience of a great number of sufferers is that they find a softer mattress more comfortable. There are many causes of back pain, and if, for example, your back pain arises from certain ligaments or the facet joints in your back, a softer mattress will allow the back part of the spine to sag or gap a little bit. This consequently takes the pressure off these structures making it more comfortable than a firmer surface.

If you are thinking of buying a new bed, take time over your selection, trying as many beds as you can by lying on them, or even sleeping on them for sufficient time to assess the level of comfort or discomfort they afford you. Experience the difference between hard and soft mattresses before committing yourself to an expensive purchase. When looking around the shops wear comfortable clothes which will allow you to bounce on the different types of beds without interfering with your comfort and assessment as to whether they feel too hard or too soft.

Don't be tempted to go out and buy an orthopaedic bed just for the sake of it, because you will be paying for the name. You can buy many beds and mattresses that are quite adequate without having that magical medical term attached to their name. If you think that you might benefit from using a firmer bed, and you can't try one out, try putting your mattress on the floor for a week. This will give you quite a good indication as to whether your back does prefer a firmer surface or not. Another way of making a firm bed is to have a board in the bed. Half-inch chipboard is ideal, but some people take a door off its hinges and use that as a useful temporary measure. The board should cover the whole length of the bed, and be wide enough for the width. If you share a double bed and your partner doesn't like the board, you can have it half width. Providing the board covers the whole width, you may find it easier if the board is in several sections for ease of handling. Place the board between the base of the bed and the mattress and not on top of the mattress and just under the sheet.

Some companies offer a service of 'made-to-measure' beds. They will make the mattress to suit your individual weight and build which some people find very comfortable.

Another type of bed which is generally very good for back pain sufferers is a water bed. As your body is supported on a mattress of water, whatever position you are in while asleep, your spine is fully supported. Being thermostatically controlled, you can have the benefit of heat as well.

SLEEPING POSITIONS

For those who suffer a lot of pain at night, it may be possible to ease this slightly by trying out a variety of different sleeping positions.

If you find that a firm mattress suits you, you may achieve greater comfort by placing a little pad in the small of your

Coping with Back Pain

back. Experiment with the size and shape of it. Try using a rolled-up towel or something similar, that can be easily adjusted. Once you have adjusted the size and shape of pad to suit you, it is often possible to make up a simple pad out of foam, covering it with material. Once made up, these little pads are also useful to carry around with you for use as a support when you are sitting.

Many people like to lie on their side to sleep, but find that this becomes uncomfortable. When lying on your side, try bending up your top leg and resting it on one or two pillows. Doing this will stop your knee dropping on to the mattress which can cause a stretching strain on one side of the spine.

For those people who prefer to lie on their backs on a softer mattress, it may be beneficial to place a pillow under your knees. This allows your back to sag a little and takes the pressure off the structures creating the pain at the back of your spine. This is achieved by allowing them to gap slightly. Lying on your side with both knees bent up achieves much the same thing.

Lying on the tummy is a position that some people find very comfortable for their lower back, but there is the possibility of creating a neck problem. Many people wake up with neck pain because of the way they've lain in bed. When you lie on your tummy there is a tendency to sleep with your head fully turned to one side, so be wary of using this as a sleeping position.

Thinking specifically of the upper part of the spine, it is important that you support your neck in order to reduce to a minimum the same stresses that affect the rest of your spine. When you sleep with only one pillow, bunch it up in the middle to make it butterfly shaped. It is your neck that needs the pillow not your head. Resting your head and neck on the pillow, pull the bottom corners around your neck and over your shoulders to give you support for your neck at the sides as well.

If you prefer to use two pillows, try crossing them over (*see*

Coping with Back Pain

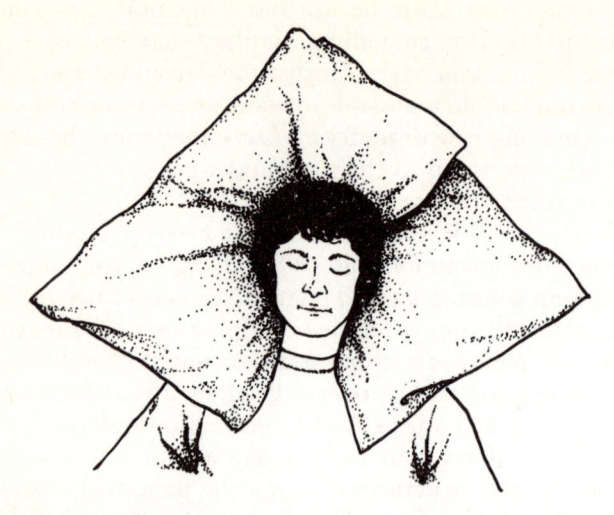

Fig 9 Crossed pillows.

Fig 9). In this way you still have the thickness of two pillows, but the extra benefit of being able to pull the corners around the sides of the neck for support.

Once you're asleep you cannot help turning over or moving, but hopefully you will be able to put yourself into a comfortable position if you should wake up in pain. After repositioning yourself you may be able to get back to sleep again more easily. Although it may sound silly, it can be very therapeutic to cuddle a teddy bear or a pillow. Many people find that holding something against the tummy helps to support their back.

When you wake up in the morning, don't jump out of bed before everything has had a chance to wake up! Sudden movements, before your body is ready, could quite easily 'tweak' something, and cause pain. When you feel you are ready to get out of bed, bend your knees up and roll on to your side, so that your lower legs are on the edge of the bed. Push up on your arms to lift your head and shoulders up and at the same time, lower your feet to the ground. You will end up sitting on the edge of the bed without having twisted your spine. You can use the reverse of this to get into bed at the end of the day.

AVOIDING THE STOOP AND THE TWIST

Bedmaking

Many people find that it is easier to maintain a comfortable back position if they make the bed while on their knees, and that squatting down and getting up to move to another part of the bed before squatting down again is uncomfortable. If, when trying this, you find that it gives you sore knees, try using some form of knee-pads. You can either buy ready-made ones or, alternatively, make up a pair of your own with two pieces of reasonably thick foam and a few pieces of wide elastic.

If the bed is normally positioned with one side against a wall, either ease the bed away from the wall to make it, enabling you to walk around it, or, if the bed can't be moved, get on to the bed on all fours. This allows you to make the bed with your spine in a straight position rather than stooping as you stand at the side of the bed and lean over to make it. It is also worth remembering that it is much easier to make the bed if you use a duvet, rather than trying to handle several layers of sheets and blankets. Because there are less layers with a duvet, it obviously follows that there will be less bending and tucking in to do.

Dressing

If you are not able to bend forward, you will find out how much of a problem getting dressed can be; for example,

Coping with Back Pain

trying to get your clothes on over your feet when your back is painful. Perhaps one of the easiest ways of getting your shoes, socks and stockings on in this situation, is to lie down on your back, bringing one foot up towards you at a time. Avoid being tempted to sit down to put them on, as by doing this you have combined the two dangerous positions of sitting and stooping. At times where it would not be practical to lie down, an alternative way of reaching your foot would be to stand up and bring your foot up towards you, perhaps resting it on a chair or a table. Another way of approaching this is to squat down to your foot, keeping your back straight.

There are now a variety of very handy 'tools', or gadgets, which, although they were perhaps originally designed to help disabled persons to dress themselves, have proved invaluable to a very wide range of users. There are long-handled shoe horns to ease the task of putting on shoes. Elastic shoe laces are available for people who prefer lace-tie shoes, with the convenience of being able to just slip them on and off.

In the Bathroom

Surprising though it may seem, the bathroom can be quite a hazardous area for back pain sufferers, if they are not aware of the possible dangers. Just stop for a moment and think of the postures that you now know you should avoid and see how you could easily put yourself into a bad posture in most bathrooms. There are quite a few people who have actually 'put their backs out' whilst leaning over the wash-basin to wash their hair, clean their teeth or just have a shave. An ideal solution is to have a shower area, where all of your toiletry requisites can be at hand and you are able to do everything standing up. If you have to use the wash-basin, try sitting down instead of standing and bending over. You can then rest your body against the edge of the basin. If you do stand up at the wash-basin, remember to stick your bottom out and pivot at the hips, keeping that natural shape in your back as you lean forward. By leaning your body weight through your arms on to the rim of the wash-basin, if it will take your weight, you will again release some of the strain from your back.

Instead of leaning over a wash-basin or sink to wash the hair, using one of the small shower attachments that just pushes on over the taps, kneel down and lean over the bath. This is often a much better position as some of the weight of your trunk is taken by the side of the bath. If you find the rim of the bath uncomfortable, lean against some form of pad, such as a folded towel.

Most people find a nice hot bath very soothing for their backache. However, they are often not able to enjoy as long a soak as they would like because the shape of the bath forces their back into a stooped posture. This becomes uncomfortable, to say the least, after only a short while. Take a tip from one of our patients. Try putting hot water bottles (filled with suitably warm water) in the curves of your lower back and neck to support your spine. A longer stay in the soothing warmth of the bath is now far more comfortable.

After your bath, unfortunately you then have to clean it. You might find it easier to clean the bath before you get out, but avoid any twisting in the process. To clean the bath from outside, preferably use a long-handled mop or broom, which will enable you to stand up whilst cleaning. You may also find putting one foot in the bath helps you to avoid leaning forward when you are doing this. Another alternative method for bath cleaning, holding a cloth in your hand, is to kneel down beside the bath and lean your trunk against it.

In the Garden

When you are weeding or planting out, do it on all fours, rather than trying to do it in any way that causes you to stoop or twist. At times you may find that you will be working in

Coping with Back Pain

the same place for some time. You may find it more comfortable to rest your trunk on the top of a padded stool. By doing this you also have both hands free when they are needed.

When hoeing or mowing, remember to apply your six 'rules'. Keeping your back in a nice upright posture, use your body weight to do most of the work by moving your feet to help avoid any twisting movements. With a hover-type lawn mower, be particularly careful not to swing it from side to side, as this motion puts a nasty shearing strain on the structures of your back. It can be easy to do this with a hover mower, so beware!

Mowing slopes can be difficult, so try to do this either by pushing the mower up the slope, if it is shallow enough, or stand at the top and manoeuvre the mower up and down the slope by using a rope securely tied to the mower. Don't be tempted to walk down steep slopes with a mower, as this will cause you to stoop.

Another gardener's tool which is very easy to stoop to use is the wheelbarrow. Whenever you are wheeling a barrow, be very conscious of your posture. To stop yourself stooping, hold the handles just behind your hips, in the same way as when carrying things. This helps you to keep upright. Our own experience has been that some of the smaller gardener's wheelbarrows have fairly short handles which make standing up and holding the handles just behind the hips difficult. The industrial type of wheelbarrow is often easier to use as it has longer handles, and with the large inflatable front tyre, doesn't seem to have the same tendency to tip over. 'Ball barrows' also seem to be more stable than those with small or thin wheels.

Remember what has already been said about the first gardening of the season; begin gently and listen to your back.

Sexual Activity

Back pain can have a stressful effect on a couple's relationship when one of the partners finds that sexual activity increases back pain, either during activity or afterwards. This can be quite distressing to both partners and considerable understanding and co-operation may be needed on both sides to try and solve the problem.

Establishing what activities bring on the pain is not always easy. If pain comes on during activity it may be possible to identify a particular movement or position that is the cause. By trying to avoid these you may well be able to eliminate much of the problem. When no pain is experienced during activity, but comes on afterwards, this makes it more difficult to determine the precise cause and to cope with it accordingly. Do not continue with anything that either partner finds painful. Understanding the needs and limitations of one's partner is essential.

You may find it helpful to use a firm surface for more support. Often, a firmly sprung mattress or a mattress without springs, such as a foam one, is beneficial. Alternatively, try placing boards under the mattress in the same way as described earlier, or perhaps use a rug or thick blanket on the floor.

Be aware of the stress put on your back when you lean forward. Try to support the weight of your trunk on your elbows, arms or hands whenever possible. Without supporting your trunk in this way, considerable strain will be put on the muscles of the back, and any movement will exaggerate this. With regard to body movement, some people find that it is the action of tilting the pelvis backwards and forwards that produces their discomfort. If you find that this is the case, the situation can often be eased by allowing the other partner to carry out most of the movement instead. Another way of overcoming this particular problem is for you to use your body weight to do the movement, instead of your back. This can be achieved by resting on your hands and knees, and moving your body weight from your knees, forward on to your hands and back on to your knees to produce the necessary movements.

Try to keep your spine in a good shape whenever possible and avoid getting yourself into awkward positions, especially any that may involve twisting of the spine, or a lot of leaning backwards. Keeping your neck in a good position is also important. Whenever possible, make sure that your neck is well supported. Avoid flicking, or holding your head backwards, especially when reaching a time of climax.

It is worth talking this over with your partner and experimenting with different positions, trying out as many combinations as are comfortable for you both. Vary between taking both an active and passive role, as you may find that one may suit your back better than the other. The following positions may help in some way, either to be followed as they are, or by being adapted in some way by you.

(1) With one partner lying on their back, the other partner positions themselves above, supporting the weight of their trunk on their knees and forearms.

(2) With the male lying on his back, the female kneels astride him facing his feet, inclining her trunk forward and supporting the weight of her trunk on her hands.

(3) The female lies on her side, with the joints of her legs comfortably bent. The male moulds himself to her shape by lying on his side behind her.

(4) With the female lying on her back, the male lies on his side facing her. By placing her nearest leg over her partner's upper thigh, he interlocks their legs by placing his upper leg over the female's furthest leg.

(5) The male sits up, perhaps supported with pillows, with his legs apart and comfortably bent. The female lies down on her back, resting her raised legs on the shoulders of her partner.

(6) Both partners sit facing each other, the male with his legs apart and comfortably bent. The female sitting on a cushion, sits between her partner's legs with her own legs resting over him.

(7) Both partners lie on their sides facing each other, with their legs bent at hips and knees. The female places one leg on either side of her partner, the lower one under his waist and the upper one over his upper thigh.

(8) The male sits on a chair with the female sitting on his lap facing each other.

(9) The female kneels on the floor, with her trunk supported on the bed or chair. The male kneels on the floor behind her.

(10) On the bed or similar raised surface, the female lays on her back with her feet resting on the floor. The male kneels or stands facing her leaning on the surface of the bed or chair with his hands.

(11) Both partners stand, with either one leaning against a wall for support.

With any positions that you try, avoid having your legs unsupported in the air. Try to support them in some way, either on your partner or perhaps on the wall or headboard. If only one partner suffers from back pain, then that partner should try to maintain the natural 'S' shape of their spine, to which their partner then conforms.

If you have the opportunity of using a private swimming pool or a large enough bath, you may find sexual activity a lot more comfortable, as the weight of your body is supported by the water.

6
Treatments Available

Because of the problems that any practitioner has in making a precise diagnosis as to which particular structure is producing the pain, planning a course of treatment can sometimes be difficult – all people are individuals, and so are their backs. Having examined a patient, the practitioner or therapist will have a good idea as to what is likely to help that particular patient and their problem. From this assessment they are able to formulate a suitable treatment plan. This treatment plan is then followed through in a logical manner, until the most effective modality is found.

Back pain does not have to be tolerated as 'one of those things' and it is not the case that having tried one type of treatment you just have to 'learn to live with it'. There are, these days, many treatments available to back pain sufferers, from both conventional and alternative medicine and most have a positive part to play in the treatment of back pain. Physiotherapy is perhaps the most widely used form of treatment and is available privately and within the NHS.

Some of the treatments available are not suitable for certain categories of patients and conditions. Wrongly applied they can create more pain, or at worst, they can be dangerous. For this reason, if you are considering visiting a private practitioner, make sure they are registered with the appropriate professional society (*see* Appendix).

TRACTION

Traction is usually given for a period of between ten and twenty minutes, either on a daily basis, or two or three times

Treatments Available

in a week. Treatment by traction can be used on any area of the spine. This is usually practised on an electrically-operated couch, by applying harnesses to whichever area of the spine is to be tractioned. If your particular problem is one of stiffness, you may be given intermittent traction. Intermittent traction is applied pulling for a chosen period of time and releasing on a rhythmical basis. This type of traction often helps to 'loosen' the spine up. If your problem is one of referred pain, you are more likely to be given static traction, where the same level of pull is maintained continuously throughout the treatment time. This type of traction can help to relieve cases where part of a disc has moved and is causing pressure to be put on nerves. It achieves this by the 'suction' effect that traction creates, encouraging the displaced piece of disc back into its normal position.

Some patients are admitted to hospital for continuous traction. This is applied by using weights which are attached to a harness either around the pelvis or the neck, with the bed tilted to use the patient's body weight as a counterforce. With continuous traction, a lower poundage of weight is applied than would be used in the type of static traction described above on an out-patient basis.

For people who do gain benefit from traction, there is an appliance for use by the patient at home. It is known as the 'backswing' and is a very effective way of tractioning either the thoracic spine, or the whole spine if you suffer with pain in more than one area. Once clamped in by your feet, you are then able to gently ease yourself backwards to the point where you can swing upside-down by altering the position of your arms. The movement of your arms alters your centre of gravity, allowing you to control exactly how far back you swing, just by slowly moving your arms above your head. You are able either to stay upside-down, which gives you a static type of traction, or, if you prefer, you can swing gently by moving your arms up and down which gives you an intermittent type of traction.

If you are considering whether or not to buy this type of equipment, it is very important that you consult with your practitioner first, whether doctor or therapist, as it may not always be suitable. Only patients with a long-standing or chronic back pain condition and benefiting from this type of treatment should consider investing in this sort of machine.

MANIPULATION AND MOBILISATION

Manipulation is the forceful movement of a joint or joints, carried out beyond the control of the patient. This means that once a manipulation technique is started, you as a patient have no control over what is being done. It is a traumatic technique and produces some tissue damage. For this reason patients should be carefully selected and the treatment should not be carried out unnecessarily. For example, if you have low back pain, this does not necessarily mean that your back needs manipulating to ease the pain. Also, you do not need to be manipulated at a time when you are pain-free.

Used in wrongly-selected patients, manipulation can be dangerous, particularly in the hands of the untrained. So make sure that the practitioner that you are visiting for consultation has some recognised form of training.

Mobilisations are a gentler form of manipulation. These techniques are carried out under the patient's control. Very gentle movements can be used to achieve pain relief. Some of these are so gentle that, as a patient, you may not be able to detect any movement. Stronger movements are employed to increase the range of a stiff joint. Mobilisations can sometimes have quite dramatic effects in the relief of pain, with occasionally only a few minutes of treatment being required. These techniques, like manipulations, can either be localised to one particular joint, or applied in such a way that they affect several joints. Each individual vertebra can be moved by applying thumb or hand pressure over appropriate areas of the spine. A more generalised movement may be made by rotating your spine with one hand on your shoulder and the other hand on your leg, or by putting a manual traction pull on either one or both of your legs. Many back problems can, and have been, very successfully treated with the gentler mobilisations, without having to resort to the more traumatic manipulation.

MASSAGE

Massage of the soft tissues around the back can often be a very effective way of relieving pain and easing muscle tension. There are many different techniques of massage, each having a different effect on the tissues to which it is applied. What you experience can be quite gentle, pleasant and relaxing, resulting in a pleasant warmth from increased blood flow and a loss of tension within the muscles. This leaves you with a general feeling of well-being. Sometimes massage can be used much more vigorously. Your muscles can become 'knotted up', often described as 'fibrositis'. In cases such as this the massage is performed quite deeply to 'break up the knots'. This can be quite uncomfortable during the massage and for a short while afterwards as well. However, when this initial soreness does wear off, the patient is often aware of considerable improvement.

For a general massage, talcum powder is sometimes used to allow the hands of the practitioner to glide smoothly over your skin. Oil can also be used, both to allow the smooth movement of hands over skin, and also for therapeutic purposes. Aromatherapy uses pure essential plant oils. These essential oils, in the hands of an experienced therapist, can benefit many conditions within the body, in addition to the benefits of massage.

Treatments Available

PULSED SHORT WAVE

A pulsed short wave machine produces an electro-magnetic field within the tissues, which promotes the body's natural healing processes. This is achieved by improving the flow of helpful chemicals within the tissues of the body. The treatment can be applied in one of two ways. First, via a large 'head' of about 6 in (16 cm) in diameter. Secondly, it can be applied through two electrodes which are placed on either side of the part that is to be treated, for example, on either side of the shoulder, or along the part to be treated, perhaps along the spine. The head or electrodes are placed close to the skin. Very little, if anything, is felt by the patient during the application of this treatment, which can last from ten to twenty minutes each session. Most of these machines are rather large, but there are now smaller versions available for suitable patients to use at home. Again it is important to consult with your practitioner to ensure that this type of equipment is suitable and effective for you, before considering whether to buy one.

ULTRASOUND

Treatment with ultrasound consists of high frequency sound waves, which are transmitted to the patient from the machine through a conducting medium, usually in the form of a jelly or water. This medium is essential, as ultrasound waves do not travel through air. Water can be more convenient when treating hands and feet, as these can be immersed, whereas jelly is more suitable for other areas of the body, such as the back. The transmitting 'head' of the machine can vary in size from about ½in (1cm) to about 1½in (3cm) in diameter. Inside the head is a quartz crystal from which the sound waves are produced.

Ultrasound is mainly used when there is a localised tender

area, for example, if you have a torn ligament in your back. It works by producing a mechanical vibration effect. This can either help to stop scar tissue forming, or breaks scar tissue down if it is already there. As a result of this very high frequency vibration, some heating effect is produced within the tissues. This heat is felt as a warmth by the patient, particularly with the higher doses. Local blood circulation is increased because of this, promoting the body's natural healing processes by bringing nutritious substances and beneficial chemicals to the area, and removing waste products and toxins. The treatment time tends to be short, five minutes being the usual dose.

INTERFERENTIAL TREATMENT

With interferential treatment two electrical currents are applied in such a way as to cross the painful area. The current is applied to the surface of the skin using four electrodes. These may be made of rubber and bandaged into place. Some are made of metal in the bottom of rubber suction cups, with a circular piece of wet foam placed into the cups to conduct the current from the electrode to the skin. The cups are fixed to the skin by suction from the machine. Little button electrodes are sometimes used if you are having a small area treated, such as a particular joint or ligament in your back. These are four tiny electrodes of about ½in (1.5cm) in diameter, covered in material and all attached to a base of approximately 2¼in (6cm) square. This is then attached to the skin with a bandage, the base being placed in such a way as to put the area to be treated in the centre of the four electrodes. At this central point the two currents cross and 'interfere' with each other, having a beneficial effect on the tissues. Depending on which frequency is chosen, different effects can be achieved, for example higher frequencies help to reduce pain.

TRANSCUTANEOUS NERVE STIMULATION

Meaning 'stimulation of the nerves through the skin', it is commonly referred to as TNS or TENS. Two or four small rubber electrodes are covered with a conducting jelly and fixed to the skin around the painful area with tape. Some people find that by varying the positions of the electrodes they are often able to achieve better effects from a TNS unit. The electrodes can be placed over or around the painful area or over acupuncture points. A lead connects each electrode to a small battery-operated machine. By switching on and adjusting the control, a pleasant tingling sensation is produced. The frequency may be altered to a fast tingling or a pulsing tingle to gain the most benefit. It varies from person to person as to which setting is most effective. How does it work? Well, when you hurt yourself, you automatically 'rub it better'. TNS works in a similar way to rubbing. It stimulates the nervous system in such a way that pain messages travelling up to the brain are stopped. When pain messages travel along the nerves, certain chemicals are released. TNS helps the body to produce different chemicals, endorphins, which are the body's own natural pain relieving substances. These endorphins help to counteract the chemicals that are present because of the pain message, and consequently help to relieve the pain.

Although these machines are very useful for treating an acute attack of pain, they are also designed to be used on a long-term basis by chronic pain sufferers. The idea is that you are 'wired up' when you get dressed in the morning, then switch the machine on when you are feeling pain. You can have it switched on twenty four hours a day if necessary. You can't 'overdose' with it. Many people find that a TNS unit controls their pain very effectively, and allows them to reduce the amount of drugs they are taking. However, these do not work for everyone, so consult your practitioner about your suitability before considering buying one. Some manufacturers operate a loan system, where you are able to try a machine for a trial period so you can see if it is suitable for your circumstances.

HYDROTHERAPY

Hydrotherapy involves exercising in a warm pool with the water usually up at around 98°F (36–37°C). The heat of the water helps to relieve pain, muscle spasm and tension. The buoyancy you gain in the water allows you to exercise more than would be safe for you on dry land.

Frequently we find that people who attend for hydrotherapy continue their treatment themselves on a regular basis at the local swimming pool. The treatments are designed to strengthen the muscles that help the functioning of your spine, and to keep the spine mobile, preventing it from stiffening up.

BACKSCHOOLS

Backschools play an important role in reducing the risk of back trouble. So, if you are someone who is painfree at the moment, attending a backschool will help you to reduce the risk of getting further trouble in the future. If you are a chronic back pain sufferer, it will teach you how to cope with your pain, and perhaps lessen the amount of pain that you experience. If you don't yet have a back pain problem, your attendance at a backschool will help you to reduce the risk of developing one.

The overall aim of a backschool is to reduce the risk of back pain by first increasing the sufferer's knowledge and understanding of the problem, secondly, by getting the

Treatments Available

sufferer to play an active role in the management of his or her own problem, and thirdly, by improving the sufferer's muscle strength and posture.

Backschools vary considerably in their content, so to give you an idea of the content of a backschool, we will describe briefly what is contained in our school which has been operating since 1981, and runs for five two-hour sessions. In the first session, after introductions and an explanation of the course, we talk about the basic structure and function of the spine, what it's made of, what can go wrong with it, and how we get various aches and pains. We then give advice on beds and relaxation positions, such as sleeping and sitting positions. Each session has a practical element, and in the first session this involves getting into the psoas position, and doing a few simple exercises designed to help relieve pain.

The second session looks at the effect of posture on back pain, and the amount of pressure put on to the spine in various activities. Simple biomechanics are used to explain the stresses exerted on the spine when we do certain handling and lifting tasks. Discussion and explanations of the six 'rules' is included. The practical part of this session involves putting the six 'rules' into practice. We do posture correction and exercises to help maintain and improve posture. There are more exercises to help relieve pain, particularly for the head and neck, and exercises to strengthen muscles to help take the strain off the back.

Session three relates the six 'rules' to everyday activities both at home and at work. Different carrying techniques are discussed and we talk about the benefits and hazards of lifting with other people. We look at different sized and shaped objects in the practical session and discuss various ways of moving and handling them.

The fourth session is everybody's favourite! We start off in the hydrotherapy pool to give people a range of exercises that they can do to help their back problems. This is followed by a session on relaxation in which patients are taught the

Treatments Available

benefits of relaxation and how to put it into practice successfully.

The final session includes advice on sports, and how to manage an acute attack of back pain, and concludes with a general discussion, revision and questions. We run through all the exercises and posture correction and show patients how to progress the exercises when appropriate.

Backschools have many proven benefits, including motivation of self-help as many patients alter their lifestyle to their benefit. Other benefits include decreased absence from work, decreased incidence and severity of pain, increased understanding by the sufferer, and probably most important of all, something that many of our patients have said, 'It's so nice to know that I'm not the only one . . .'.

Backschools held within the National Health Service are presently only available to patients already suffering from back pain, but we strongly believe that the sort of information contained in a backschool should be available to every member of the population. At the end of every school, patients always say: 'If only I'd known this before I hurt my back'. To this end we now run a backschool along the lines of an evening class. Anyone can come, and we hope to attract people who do not yet suffer, to try and help them reduce the risk of becoming another statistic. But as yet, everyone who has attended the school has already had a problem. People always think 'It won't happen to me', and it's not until they suffer pain that they realise just what a problem it is.

EXERCISES

In the treatment of back pain, there are three main types of exercise likely to benefit your spine. These are mobility exercises, strengthening exercises and relaxation exercises. It is not necessary to exercise until you are out of breath, or approaching a pain barrier, to keep your back fit. In fact you are more likely to create or worsen a back problem by exercising in that way.

The types of exercise normally given by your practitioner are gentle, and specifically designed to benefit the function of your spine. Not all these exercises are suitable for everyone, and if any exercise generates or worsens your back pain, then that particular exercise should be avoided. This advice holds strong in whatever activity you prefer to involve yourself.

Mobility Exercises

These are gentle exercises designed to keep the spine mobile. By using these you help stop your back becoming stiff. They are also very useful in helping to loosen you up if your back is already stiff.

Strengthening Exercises

Certain muscle groups are particularly beneficial in assisting the function of the spine. It is important to maintain their good strength by regularly exercising them.

Relaxation Exercises

Some exercises are designed to relax your muscles and to reduce muscle tension. This may sound like a contradiction, but by exercising in a particular way, you can help to reduce pain and much of the stress that is put on to the spine.

POSTURE CORRECTION

Bad posture involves a general slouch of the body, resulting in the spine being stooped forward. In this position, your head will be stooped, looking at the floor, so to compensate for this the head tends to poke forward to enable you to see in

Treatments Available

front of you. As a result you develop what is known as a 'poking chin deformity', which often results in a 'dowager's hump' where the neck joins on to the rest of the spine. This can give rise to aches and pains in the neck and across the tops of the shoulders. It can also cause a tension headache, where the pain radiates from the neck, up the back of the head and over the forehead. This type of pain can also be the result of deskwork, if you are sitting with your spine stooped and slouched over your work. This is pain directly related to posture.

If you do have bad posture, your muscles have to work continuously to keep you upright. This involves unnecessary use of energy, making you feel quite tired by the end of the day. Whenever a muscle is working, it contracts, and as the muscles around the spine contract and shorten, there is increased pressure put on the structures of your spine. This increases the wearing-out process of the spine, and also increases any pain that you may be experiencing.

To correct your posture, try standing with your back against a wall, and imagine you have a hook screwed into the top of your head, which is pulling you up straight. With your feet comfortably apart and your weight evenly balanced between your feet, make sure that your head is up and your chin tucked gently in. Pull your shoulders back, and tilt your pelvis backwards slightly, allowing you to feel some tension in your tummy muscles. Keeping a certain amount of tension in your tummy muscles is very useful because all the time your abdominal muscles are working, so is your abdominal balloon. This will help to take some of the stress from your spine, whether sitting, standing or walking.

If you are now standing correctly, you should feel the following areas of your body touching the wall: the back of your head; your shoulder blades; your buttocks; and possibly your calves and heels, depending on your shape. Now stand away from the wall and try the same thing again. The only muscles you should feel working continuously are your

Treatments Available

tummy muscles. The rest of you should be quite relaxed. Many people who experience pain when standing or walking have found this posture correction to be very helpful.

When you are correcting your posture, it is useful to stand naked in front of a mirror, so that you can see which parts of your body need to be worked on. To correct your posture you do, quite literally, have to keep reminding yourself, whenever you think of it, to perhaps 'keep my shoulders back' or 'hold my tummy in'. You won't be able to correct your posture overnight, it will take a lot of effort and time on your part. When you first start you may well experience increased aches and pains. For example, if you suffer from round shoulders, when you start to correct your posture, and pull your shoulders back, you will stretch the structures across the front of your chest which have become accustomed to being in a shortened position. The muscles between your shoulder blades may start to ache as well, as they will have to start doing work that they are not used to. But don't give up, these aches will go away if you persevere, and you will end up with all the benefits of a better posture.

RELAXATION

When you have pain, your body's natural reaction is for your muscles to tense up. In tensing up, the muscles put more pressure on the structures producing the pain, which in turn produces more pain. As the muscle tension is increased in response to this increased pain, a vicious circle is being set up. By learning physically to relax the muscles, you will break into this circle, and as a consequence, reduce the amount of pain that is being created.

Do remember that by relaxing you can help to reduce both pain and the wearing-out process of your spine. Try to put by a period of time each day in which to relax properly. Choose a time when you will not be interrupted; make sure that you

Treatments Available

are wearing loose and comfortable clothing, and that the room is warm and quiet. Once you have learnt how to relax properly, you could perhaps use your ten minutes lying in the psoas position. Ideally, you should allow yourself sufficient time to relax completely, working through a sequence of relaxation, or 'letting-go' exercises. These enable you to relax all the muscles in your body. Having completed a sequence of 'letting-go' exercises, you can then utilise your own breathing pattern to deepen the relaxation. When you achieve a feeling of deep relaxation, it is beneficial to build up a pleasant, relaxing scene in your mind. This is very important, as you cannot truly relax your body, without relaxing your mind as well.

There are times during a normal day when it is impossible to remain calm and relaxed, and you may become aware of tension in some parts of your body. As you become more experienced at relaxation, you will be able to recognise easily if different parts of your body are tense or relaxed. To begin with, try thinking about different muscles from time to time, and just feel whether they are tense or relaxed. Should they feel tense, consciously try to relax them. Just think for a moment about the muscles across the top of your shoulders. Are they completely relaxed, or can you 'let go' a bit more, and as you do can you feel the tension lessening? Be aware of the muscles in your face; are you frowning, squinting or clenching your jaw? If you feel you are doing any of these, 'let go', and feel the muscles relax. If you are someone who finds it difficult to just 'let go', try to tighten up the muscles as hard as you can first, and then 'let go'. As you become more practised at this, you will be able to tell the difference between tensed and relaxed muscles much easier. Just allow yourself to become aware of any tension as it develops, and release it before it begins to give you pain. If you are interested in developing your ability to relax, you may find a recorded relaxation session helpful (*see* page 96).

Treatments Available

ACUPUNCTURE

Thousands of years ago someone noticed that warriors who had been wounded with arrows were becoming cured of various diseases from which they had been suffering. This was the beginning of the existence of acupuncture, probably about four thousand years ago. Acupuncture has a recorded history of two thousand years. It was discovered that certain points on the body were associated with a particular organ or system. When that organ or system became diseased, the points associated with it became tender, and if these points were 'needled', the disease could be cured. All the points associated with a particular organ or system were joined up to form meridians.

In traditional acupuncture there is said to be a life force called 'chi' or 'Qi' which flows along the meridians much like blood flows through our blood vessels. The chi is made up of 'yin' and 'yang' which are two opposing forces. For a state of health to exist, there must be a balance between the yin and the yang. If these become unbalanced, disease occurs. Acupuncture points are chosen to re-balance the yin and yang and cure the disease.

Acupuncture for the relief of pain is available within the National Health Service, in some physiotherapy clinics and pain relief clinics. The number of hospitals providing this service is growing.

If you visit an acupuncturist outside the National Health Service do make sure that they have a recognised qualification (*see* Appendix). It is also advisable to ensure that either autoclaved or disposable needles are being used, otherwise there is a risk that infectious diseases can be transmitted from one patient to another. It is for this reason that if you are a blood donor, you are asked not to donate blood if you have had acupuncture, unless it was within the National Health Service.

Research into acupuncture has shown that certain

Treatments Available

chemicals are released both during and after acupuncture. These chemicals have a useful effect on our nervous system by blocking out the pain messages travelling along the nerves. They are called endorphins and are the body's own natural morphine-like pain relievers. Acupuncture can be applied in many different ways.

Draining is a technique in which the needles are inserted into tender acupuncture points and left *in situ* for about twenty minutes. For back pain, needles are likely to be placed along the spine and down the arms and legs. Sometimes putting a needle in the foot can be used to treat for example, neck pain, as the meridian that passes over the painful area in the neck runs down the back and leg. Therefore a needle put into a point on the leg can have an effect in relieving pain in the neck.

Supplying is a 'stronger' form of acupuncture, and can be achieved by manually 'twiddling' the needles, or by attaching an electro-acupuncture machine to the needles with leads and clips. Manually, the needles are usually supplied for thirty seconds to a minute, then removed, sometimes being left in for twenty minutes and supplied for thirty seconds at a time during this period. With electro-acupuncture, the needles are supplied for twenty minutes.

Once the needle is inserted in a point, a 'needling sensation' or 'dequi' is sometimes felt by the patient, around, and sometimes radiating away from, the needle. This can be felt as an ache, tingling, heaviness, numbness and various other sensations, varying from person to person. These sensations are usually a sign that the treatment is likely to be effective.

The term 'moxibustion' means 'to scar with a burning object', and some years ago this was literally true. Nowadays the heat is applied without producing any scarring. This heat may be generated in a variety of ways from the burning of herbs on the needle handle, to heating the handle of the needle with a lighter. The technique is particularly useful in the treatment of pain arising from arthritic joints.

Treatments Available

EAR ACUPUNCTURE

Also known as Auriculotherapy or Auricular Acupuncture, this involves putting needles into acupuncture points in the ears. This was developed in the mid-nineteenth century by a Frenchman named Nogier who likened the ear to an inverted foetus, with the head being represented by the ear lobe. Every part of the body is represented on the ear, and the points are named after the parts of the body they represent.

Usually, two needles are inserted into points corresponding to where the patient is feeling the pain, and the electro-acupuncture machine is attached for a twenty-minute treatment.

With patients who have chronic pain, a 'stud' may be inserted into an acupuncture point, fixed in with strong tape, and left *in situ* for a week. All the time it is in place, it is helping to produce pain relief by releasing endorphins. If the patient has an increase in pain, they 'twiddle' the needle between their thumb and finger, producing an increased flow of endorphins to help produce better pain relief. Some people find that they are able to reduce the amount of drugs they are taking by using a stud.

ACUPRESSURE

Also known as 'shiatsu', this involves massaging the acupuncture points. Patients who are undergoing acupuncture can sometimes use acupressure on themselves at home, between treatments, to help relieve pain.

MEDICATION

There are four main types of drug available to help the back pain sufferer: painkillers or analgesics; anti-inflammatories;

muscle relaxants; anti-depressants. Whichever type of medication you are taking, it is important to take your drugs as prescribed by your doctor. In the event of them not helping you, or causing you any problems, it is important to inform your doctor, as there are many different types of the same drug available. Where one type of drug may not help you, another type might. Some of these drugs may give rise to certain side effects, others will not. So consult your physician and talk over the problems.

Analgesics

Some examples of commonly used analgesics are:

Paracetamol	DF 118	Coproxamol
Codeine	Distalgesic	Panadol

The objective of a painkiller is to do just what it says, kill pain. You do have to be careful when you are taking a painkiller not to overdo it. Always remember that pain is your warning signal that something is wrong with you. When you block out the pain with a drug, the damage is still present, but you just can't feel it. If you are not careful, you may do something that will cause even more damage. The painkiller will make you feel more comfortable, but it will not cure your back problem. Do remember that you should always consult your doctor for advice when you develop pain of any description.

Anti-Inflammatories

Some of the most commonly used anti-inflammatories are:

Aspirin	Voltarol	Codis	Indocid
Nurofen	Brufen	Feldene	Naprosyn

Treatments Available

Inflammation of the tissues occurs when you have 'arthritis' in your back, or when you damage it, perhaps by tearing a muscle or ligament. The inflamed part becomes hot, red and swollen, creating pain. Anti-inflammatory drugs help to reduce this inflammation by getting at the seat of the trouble. By reducing the inflammation, your pain is also reduced. To enable this type of medication to have a full effect, it must be taken regularly, as prescribed, in a course of treatment. These drugs are unlikely to be as effective if you just take them occasionally, when you have pain, in the way you would take a painkiller.

One of the possible side effects of this type of drug is to cause irritation to the stomach wall. If you should develop any nausea, stomach pains or indigestion, tell your doctor so that he can change your drug if necessary. These drugs are most commonly taken in tablet form or as a liquid. When they do cause stomach upsets, they can also be taken as a suppository, which helps to reduce the unpleasant side effects.

Muscle Relaxants

Some of the popular muscle relaxant drugs in common use are Robaxin, Norflex, Lobak and Valium. The action of this type of medication is to help reduce the level of muscle spasm and tension that occurs when you either damage yourself, or are in pain. By helping the affected muscles to relax, any pain that you are experiencing, which is due to tension in your muscles, will be reduced. This muscle spasm can create quite a lot of pain, so the muscle relaxant is sometimes a very useful drug to the sufferer of back pain.

Anti-Depressants

One example of an anti-depressant is Amitryptiline. This type of medication is not necessarily given to you because your doctor thinks you are depressed. The reason is quite likely to be that because of the way these drugs work chemically within the body, they can have a very useful effect in helping to control pain. It is often for this reason that anti-depressants are prescribed as painkillers.

LOCAL STEROID INJECTIONS

This style of treatment is sometimes used for people who have a localised tender spot, for example, having torn one of the ligaments between two of your vertebrae. In these cases, injecting this area with an anti-inflammatory substance, such as hydrocortisone, can prove to be very effective. A local anaesthetic is often injected with the anti-inflammatory, as this helps ease the pain that can be associated with this type of injection. After any initial pain or discomfort has worn off, there can be a total relief of pain for up to three weeks afterwards. Sometimes the pain relief from this type of treatment is only temporary, in which case it may be advisable to have another injection. Some general practitioners will give this type of injection themselves while others will refer their patients to a hospital consultant.

EPIDURAL

If you are suffering from nerve root pain, an epidural injection may help to ease it. If a structure such as a torn disc is irritating a nerve it will become inflamed around the site of irritation. It is this type of irritation that gives rise to referred pain. There are occasions when the original cause of the pain has long since gone (with the torn disc it may have moved back to its natural position), but the pain still remains. This is because the inflammation around the nerve is still there.

To settle this inflammation, anti-inflammatory drugs may

be all that is necessary, but if these do not work an epidural injection may be considered. This treatment involves injecting an anti-inflammatory substance together with a local anaesthetic, into the epidural space, which is a fluid filled space around the spinal cord. This injection is carried out under sterile conditions in an operating theatre. Immediately after receiving this injection, you feel numbness in the areas below the site of injection. As an example, if the injection is made in the lower back, for leg pain, you will experience numbness from the waist down. This numbness will gradually turn to a feeling of pins and needles and within a few hours your normal sensation will return. In many cases this technique is applied on an out-patient basis, involving about half a day. It is worth noting that an epidural can take up to three weeks to have its full effect and that you may find that you need more than one to settle your condition.

FACET JOINT INJECTIONS

Sometimes it can be one or more of the little facet joints in your back causing the pain that you are experiencing. When this is suspected, to confirm whether a particular joint is causing pain, it can be injected with a local anaesthetic. If the pain goes away, this will confirm that it is that particular joint responsible for your problem. On occasions it will only require an injection of local anaesthetic into the joint to stop the pain. In other cases it may be found necessary to inject the joint with an anti-inflammatory substance as well.

To facilitate facet joint injections, the procedure is carried out under sterile conditions in the X-ray department, as this enables the doctor to monitor the joint and see exactly where he is injecting on the screen. Under normal circumstances this type of treatment is also carried out on an out-patient basis.

Treatments Available

NERVE BLOCKS

The reason that any of us feel pain is because of the electrical impulses travelling along our nerves. In certain conditions these impulses can keep on firing for no good reason after the original cause of the pain has gone away. When this happens it can give rise to constant pain being experienced. When this situation exists, the nerve can be 'blocked' to stop the pain impulses. In sterile conditions, the responsible nerve is destroyed, either with heat or cold, preventing it from transmitting any further pain. A local anaesthetic is used in order to make the procedure more comfortable and is again normally done on an out-patient basis.

HYPNOTHERAPY

The use of hypnosis in the relief of pain has become much more widely used in the last few years. The state of hypnosis is a natural phenomenon, which anyone can experience. There is no magic, it is a natural altered state of consciousness and each one of us pass through the hypnotic state at least twice a day; when going off to sleep and when we wake up. It is best described as that pleasant feeling of being half asleep; totally aware of what is going on around you, but not wanting, or bothering to open your eyes.

The role of the hypnotherapist is to enhance abilities already within you. It is you who elects to enter the hypnotic state and the hypnotherapist only assists you in the process. All of us have the power to imagine and the therapist can invite you to imagine perhaps that your body is feeling comfortable and relaxed. This introduction into the hypnotic state is called the induction. Once you are fully relaxed and in the hypnotic state, it becomes much easier to achieve control over the pain. Your therapist is able to make helpful suggestions to you as to how you are able to achieve this.

Treatments Available

Whilst you are in the hypnotic state, you are fully aware of what is happening around you and the therapist has no hold or power over you whatsoever, if you do not wish to cooperate during the session. There is no way that you can be made to do anything that you would not normally do and you can come out of the hypnotic state if you wish.

Once you have experienced a few sessions of hypnotherapy, the therapist can teach you how to achieve this state for yourself at home. This is called self-hypnosis because you induce the hypnotic state yourself; and when you are ready, you bring the session to an end, coming out of your hypnotic state on your own. Some people find this easier to achieve than others. With practice you can achieve a deep state of hypnosis, using it to help control your pain. Like learning any new skill, it takes a lot of effort and concentration to start with, but with practice it becomes almost automatic when you wish to use it.

Hypnosis is not a magic cure for pain, but it can be a very effective aid for people with chronic back pain, helping them to cope with it.

SURGERY

Surgical operations on the spine are not undertaken lightly. They will normally only be considered if all of the more conservative methods of treatment have failed. One very relevant reason for this is that following an initial period of relief from pain, after surgery, the pain can return. This can often be due to a build up of scar tissue, especially around the nerves. Once this has occurred, there is little that can be done for you, as further surgery would only produce more scar tissue. In trying to prevent this happening, certain exercises should be done after the operation.

Prior to surgery, a myelogram or radiculogram is often carried out. These procedures are undertaken in the X-ray department, and involve a dye being injected into the area around the discs and nerves. This dye shows up on the X-ray film and enables the surgeon to see whether part of the disc has moved from its normal position, or whether there is any pressure on the nerve roots. By using this procedure it is also possible to confirm which particular disc or nerve is involved.

LAMINECTOMY

This means the removal of part of the vertebra, 'ectomy' meaning removal, and 'lamina' being part of the vertebra. This type of operation is often offered to people who have a damaged disc pressing on the nerves. During the operation the loose parts of the disc are removed, together with little pieces of bone from the vertebra. This takes the pressure off the nerves and allows them plenty of room.

FUSION

Another form of surgery that can be carried out, if a large amount of bone has to be removed during the operation, is fusion. A fusion is carried out to stabilise the remaining structures, ensuring there is no excessive movement. This procedure involves taking bone, usually from the pelvis, and then grafting it into the unstable vertebrae.

REST

You may have decided to rest to help your back, or, if you have consulted your doctor, you may have been told to rest at home. Although this is often termed 'bed rest', it does not necessarily mean that you have to be in bed. The important

Treatments Available

thing is that you remain in a horizontal position, thereby taking all the pressure off the spinal structures. It doesn't really matter where; in bed, in the garden, or on the lounge floor. Try to use the psoas position, if you can get into it, as this will probably relieve much of your pain (Fig 8). Put your legs up on a stool, coffee table, a chair or any other similar raised area where you are able to have your lower legs comfortably supported. Have them resting on something soft, such as a cushion, as hard surfaces tend to interfere with the circulation within the legs, and you may then get numb feet. Try varying the height at which your legs are supported, as you will find some levels are more comfortable than others. By moving your body closer to, or further away, from the leg support, you will find the most comfortable angle at the hips for you. You may also find that some kind of support in the curve of your lower back is helpful. Try a foam pad, rolled-up towel or a warm hot water bottle. Experiment with different angles at the hips, and different shapes and sizes of support, until you find the position and support that suits you best. Some similar form of support for the curve of the neck can also prove beneficial to some people.

If you rest properly at the first signs of back pain developing, you stand a very good chance that it will settle down quite quickly. However, if you do not have true bed rest, then you may well find the problem will linger on for weeks or possibly even months.

HEAT AND ICE

Probably the best forms of heat to use within the home are the hot water bottle and the hot bath. Do make sure that the heat is a comfortable temperature; the term 'hot' in these situations is not meant to mean hot enough to burn or cause discomfort. Hot water bottles are generally best covered before placing them over the painful area. It can also prove to be a very effective cushion for supporting the lower back, the neck, or both if you use two, at the same time giving the benefits of heat to the painful area.

Ice packs can often be very effective in the treatment of pain. For use in the home, the best way to make an ice pack is to buy a bag of frozen peas. Keep them in the freezer, and when required, take the bag out and wrap it in a tea towel. Place this pack over the painful area for ten minutes. After your treatment, take the bag of peas out of the towel and put it back into the freezer for next time.

SUMMARY

In this book we have endeavoured to give an introduction to a subject which affects a very large proportion of the population. It is quite possible that you may have only experienced minor twinges and have read this book more out of interest than serious concern. On the other hand it is possible that you may be searching in absolute desperation for some way of finding relief for a long-standing severe condition. Either way, this practical guide to coping with back pain will hopefully be of benefit to you. Remember how complicated a structure your back is, with the various different structures all at risk of being damaged or irritated.

To gain the maximum benefit may take considerable effort, as you may find that you are trying to change the habits of a lifetime. Experience has shown that if you are able to persevere with thinking about what you are doing and how you are treating your back, then the chances of creating a severe back pain problem, or aggravating the one you already have, are considerably reduced. We wish you well in your endeavours.

Appendix – Useful Addresses

The British Acupuncture Association
8 Hunter Street
London WC1N 1BN

The Chartered Society of Physiotherapy
14 Bedford Row
London WC12 4ED

General Council and Register of Osteopaths
21 Suffolk Street
London SW1Y 4HG

British Chiropractic Association
10 Greycoat Place
London SW1P 1SB

National Back Pain Association
31–33 Park Road
Teddington
Middlesex TW11 0AB

Linda and David Tagg
Back To Work
PO Box 67
Basingstoke
Hants RG24 0YG

(Write for details of a relaxation and exercise tape produced by the authors.)